Acing the USMLE and the Match
A Guide for International Medical Graduates

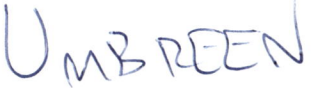

Note

This is the first edition of the book and wherever you may be and whatever stage you are in, we welcome you to send us your contributions and suggestions or just about anything you feel will help someone in your shoes. If you would like the readers of the book to hear your experience with the match, or if you have letters of recommendation or personal statements, which you would like to get published, e-mail us at acingtheusmle@gmail.com. All contributions will be duly acknowledged.

If you have any questions or doubts about the book, please e-mail us at acingtheusmle@gmail.com or e-mail the contributors of the chapters and we will do our best to reply as soon as possible.

Acing the USMLE and the Match
A Guide for International Medical Graduates

Editor
Muralikrishna Gopal MD
Resident, Department of Internal Medicine
University of Texas Medical Branch (UTMB)
Galveston, TX 77550 USA
e-mail: krishna1033@yahoo.com

Associate Editor
Paari Murugan MD
Resident, Department of Pathology
Jawaharlal Institute of Postgraduate
Medical Education and Research (JIPMER)
Pondicherry – 605006, India
e-mail: paaricmc@gmail.com

Co-editors
Nirav Mamdani MD
MP Shah Medical College
Jamnagar, Gujarat, India Residency in
Internal Medicine at Wayne State University
Detroit, MI (2002-2005) Fellowship in Cardiology
at the Loma Linda University Medical Center (2005-2008)
nmamdani@ahs.llumc.edu

Jayashree Sundararajan MD
Sri Ramachandra Medical College
Chennai, India Residency in Neurology at University of
Kansas Medical Center, Kansas, MO (2006-2010) jayasree.s@gmail.com

Vijayprasad Gopichandran MD
Resident, Department of Community Health
Christian Medical College (CMC)
Vellore 632004, India

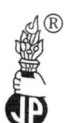

JAYPEE BROTHERS MEDICAL PUBLISHERS (P) LTD
New Delhi • Ahmedabad • Bengaluru • Chennai • Hyderabad • Kochi • Kolkata
• Lucknow • Mumbai • Nagpur

Published by
Jitendar P Vij
Jaypee Brothers Medical Publishers (P) Ltd
B-3 EMCA House, 23/23B Ansari Road, Daryaganj, **New Delhi** 110 002, India
Phones: +91-11-23272143, +91-11-23272703, +91-11-23282021
+91-11-23245672, Rel: +91-11-32558559   Fax: +91-11-23276490
+91-11-23245683, e-mail: jaypee@jaypeebrothers.com
Visit our website: www.jaypeebrothers.com

Branches

- 2/B, Akruti Society, Jodhpur Gam Road Satellite
  Ahmedabad 380 015   Phones: +91-79-26926233, Rel: +91-79-32988717
  Fax: +91-79-26927094 e-mail: ahmedabad@jaypeebrothers.com
- 202 Batavia Chambers, 8 Kumara Krupa Road, Kumara Park East
  Bengaluru 560 001   Phones: +91-80-22285971, +91-80-22382956, 080-22372664
  Rel: +91-80-32714073   Fax: +91-80-22281761
  e-mail: bangalore@jaypeebrothers.com
- 282 IIIrd Floor, Khaleel Shirazi Estate, Fountain Plaza, Pantheon Road
  Chennai 600 008, Phones: +91-44-28193265, +91-44-28194897
  Rel: +91-44-32972089   Fax: +91-44-28193231, e-mail:chennai@jaypeebrothers.com
- 4-2-1067/1-3, 1st Floor, Balaji Building, Ramkote, Cross Road,
  Hyderabad 500 095   Phones: +91-40-66610020, +91-40-24758498,
  Rel: +91-40-32940929   Fax:+91-40-24758499,
  e-mail: hyderabad@jaypeebrothers.com
- Kuruvi Building, 1st Floor, Plot/Door No. 41/3098, B & B1, St. Vincent Road
  Kochi 682 018 Kerala   Phones: +91-484-4036109, +91-484-2395739
  +91-484-2395740   e-mail: kochi@jaypeebrothers.com
- 1-A Indian Mirror Street, Wellington Square
  Kolkata 700 013   Phones: +91-33-22651926, +91-33-22276404, +91-33-22276415
  Rel: +91-33-32901926   Fax: +91-33-22656075
  e-mail: kolkata@jaypeebrothers.com
- Lekhraj Market III, B-2, Sector-4, Faizabad Road, Indira Nagar
  Lucknow 226 016   Phones: +91-522-3040553, +91-522-3040554
  e-mail: lucknow@jaypeebrothers.com
- 106 Amit Industrial Estate, 61 Dr SS Rao Road, Near MGM Hospital, Parel
  Mumbai 400 012   Phones: +91-22-24124863, +91-22-24104532
  Rel: +91-22-32926896   Fax: +91-22-24160828, e-mail: mumbai@jaypeebrothers.com
- "KAMALPUSHPA" 38, Reshimbag, Opp. Mohota Science College, Umred Road
  Nagpur 440 009 Phone: Rel: +91-712-3245220, Fax: +91-712-2704275
  e-mail: nagpur@jaypeebrothers.com

Acing the USMLE and the Match

© 2008, Jaypee Brothers Medical Publishers

All rights reserved. No part of this publication should be reproduced, stored in a retrieval system, or transmitted in any form or by any means: electronic, mechanical, photocopying, recording, or otherwise, without the prior written permission of the editors and the publisher.

> This book has been published in good faith that the material provided by contributors is original. Every effort is made to ensure accuracy of material, but the publisher, printer and editors will not be held responsible for any inadvertent error(s). In case of any dispute, all legal matters are to be settled under Delhi jurisdiction only.

First Edition: **2008**
ISBN 978-81-8448-343-7

Typeset at   JPBMP typesetting unit
Printed at   Rajkamal Electric Press, B-35/9, G.T. Karnal Road, Delhi-110 033

Contributors

Aditi Malik
Government Medical College, Patiala, India Masters in Public Health at George Washington University, Washington DC Residency in Psychiatry at St. Elizabeth's Hospital, Washington DC (2004-2008)
aditimalik@yahoo.com

Archana Bhaskaran
Madras Medical College, Chennai, India Residency in Internal Medicine at the University of Texas Medical Branch (UTMB), Galveston, TX (2006-2009)
archanabhaskaran@yahoo.co.in

Baraa Allaf M
University of Aleppo School of Medicine, Syria Residency in Obstetrics and Gynecology at the State University of New York at Buffalo, NY (2006-2010)
baraa_allaf@yahoo.com

Chandrasekhar Yangalasetty
Guntur Medical College, Guntur, India DNB (Diplomate of National Board in Pediatrics) 1999 Residency in Pediatrics at Woodhull Medical and Mental Health Centre NY (2005-2008)
vyseerx@yahoo.co.in

Dhinager Nandagopal
Madras Medical College, Chennai, India Residency in Internal Medicine at Interfaith Medical Center, NY (2006-2009) docdhina@gmail.com

Disha Uttam Shah
Baroda Medical College, Gujarat, India Residency in Preliminary Internal Medicine at Resurrection Westlake Hospital, IL (2006-2007) Residency in Neurology at Cleveland Clinic Florida (2007-2010)

Jayashree Sundararajan
Sri Ramachandra Medical College, Chennai, India Residency in Neurology at University of Kansas Medical Center, Kansas MO (2006-2010)
jayasree.s@gmail.com

Mohanakrishnan G
Stanley Medical College, Chennai India
Junior House Officer in Redcliffe Hospital, Queensland, Australia
doc_gmk@yahoo.com

Muralikrishna Gopal
Madras Medical College, Chennai, India Residency in Internal Medicine at the University of Texas Medical Branch (UTMB),
Galveston, TX (2006-2009)
krishna1033@yahoo.com

Nirav Mamdani
MP Shah Medical College, Jamnagar, Gujarat, India Residency in Internal Medicine at Wayne State University, Detroit, MI (2002-2005)
Fellowship in Cardiology at the Loma Linda University Medical Center (2005-2008)
nmamdani@ahs.llumc.edu

Paari Murugan
Madras Medical College, Chennai, India Residency in Pathology at the Jawaharlal Institute of Postgraduate Medical Education and Research (JIPMER)
Pondicherry
India (2005-2008)
paaricmc@yahoo.com

Pragatheeswar Thirunavukkarasu
Madras Medical College, Chennai, India
Residency in Preliminary Surgery at the
Hospital of the University of
Pennsylvania (2006-2007)
pragatheeshwart@yahoo.com

Vandana Panda Goyle
Government Medical College, Patiala,
India Residency in Family Medicine at
Texas Tech University
Odessa, TX
dr_vandana2000@yahoo.co.in

Varun Agarwal
Jawaharlal Institute of Postgraduate
Medical Education and Research
(JIPMER), Pondicherry, India MS
Biology, Georgia State University (2004-2005) Residency in Internal Medicine at
William Beaumont Hospital, Royal Oak,
MI (2005-2008)
varunagrawal@yahoo.com

Vijayprasad Gopichandran
Resident, Department of Community
Health, Christian Medical College (CMC),
Vellore 632004, India

Preface

"indriyebhyah param mano manasah sattvam uttamam sattvad adhi mahan atma mahato vyaktam uttamam" (Sanskrit verse from Katha Upanisad 6.7) (Translation in English: Beyond the senses is the mind, and beyond the mind is reason, its essence. Beyond reason is the Spirit in man and beyond this is the Spirit of the Universe, the evolver of all)

The Sanskrit verse above, from the *Katha Upanishad* has two words in the verse that symbolize what this book is all about, 'Human Spirit' and 'Evolution' (Survival of the Fittest). The match every year that decides whether one gets into a US residency is essentially an analogy of the Evolutionary process where the fittest are selected and the others "deselected".

Getting into a residency in the United States is a difficult, time-consuming, multi- steps process that is financially draining too. If you make it, the reward at the end is worth the effort. And please note that this "if" is a big "IF"!

What are the credentials that Program Directors look for in applications to invite you for an interview? How many programs should one apply to? Where all Should one apply? Should one go for a J1 an H-1B visa? Should one take the pre-match or go for the match? These and many more unanswered questions are answered in this book, which the authors hope will provide a comprehensive view of the difficult path of getting into a residency training in the United States.

Other than USMLE scores, overall weight of the application and Research/ United States Clinical Experience (USCE) have emerged as important factors in the application process. This book devotes two full chapters to these two factors and would help you get a head start in the Residency application process.

The authors and contributing writers come from varied backgrounds and circumstances united by the common dream of undergoing medical specialty training in the United States. Their lives range from the common medico struggling through the drudgeries of medical school to the extraordinary that outshine all others among the peers and you can find a reflection of yourself somewhere along this book. It has been written almost entirely by International Medical Graduates who are all in different stages of getting into a US residency, Just Like You most of who have successfully gotten into a residency. None of the authors are the "superstars" of residency, those in ultra-competitive specialties or in Ivy-league programs. They are all typical IMGs, just like you and me, and hence their perspective about getting into a US residency is as real as it can be.

We hope that this book acts like the friendly seniors in college (through it can never claim to substitute the real heroes and role models) who take you under their wings and guide you through this painstaking process of applying and getting into a United States Residency.

All the best in your endeavor to get into a residency in the US

Muralikrishna Gopal

Acknowledgements

- Mr Tarun Duneja, General Manager (Publishing), M/s Jaypee Brothers Medical Publishers (Pvt.) Ltd., New Delhi and Mr Jayanandan (Chennai Branch).
- April L. McVey MD, Program Director and Associate Professor, Department of Neurology, University of Kansas Medical Center.
- Dr V Murugan, D Litt, Reader, Department of English, Presidency College, Madras University.
- All Step 3 USMLE takers who helped in compiling Chapter 8.

Abbreviations

USMLE	United State Medical Licensing Examination
MBBS	Bachelor of Medicine, Bachelor of Surgery
US	United States
PLAB	Professional Linguistic Assessment Board
OSCE	Objective Structured Clinical Examination
UK	United Kingdom
IMG	International Medical Graduate
FMG	Foreign Medical Graduate
AMG	American Medical Graduate
ERAS	Electronic Residency Application Service
ECFMG	Educational Commission for Foreign Medical Graduates
NRMP	National Resident Matching Program
FSMB	Federation of State Medical Boards
NBME	National Board of Medical Examiners
IMED	International Medical Education Directory
FAIMER	Foundation for Advancement of International Medical Education and Research
IWA	Interactive Web Application
GRE	Graduate Record Examination
TOEFL	Test of English as a Foreign Language
CCS	Computerized Case Simulation
MCQ	Multiple Choice Questions
BRS	Board Review Series
BS	Behavioral Sciences
NMS	National Medical Series
Step 2 CK	Clinical knowledge
Step 2 CS	Clinical Skills
CMDT	Comprehensive Medical Diagnosis and Treatment
ALERT	Appleton and Lange Review
DG	Data Gathering
SEP	Spoken English Proficiency
CIPS	Communication and Interpersonal Skills
FA	First Aid
UW	Usmle World
OASIS	On-line Applicant Status and Information System

S P	Standardized Patient
ICE	Integrated Clinical Encounter
PN	Patient Note
GMAT	The Graduate Management Admission Test
HDFC	Housing Development Finance Corporation
PD	Program Director
USCE	United States Clinical Experience
CV	Curriculum Vitae
HIPAA	Health Insurance Portability and Accountability Act
BMJ	British Medical Journal
EEC	Extramural Electives Compendium
LCME	Liaison Committee on Medical Education
SUNY	State University of New York
ACGME	Accreditation Council for Graduate Medical Education
LOR	Letter of Recommendation
FREIDA	Fellowship and Residency Electronic Interactive Database
AMA	American Medical Association
CAF	Common Application Form
ADTS	Applicant Document and Tracking System
MSPE	Medical Student Performance Evaluation
MKSAP	Medical Knowledge Self-Assessment Program
EAD	Employment Authorization Document
CREOG	Council on Resident Education in OBGYN
ITE	In-Training Examination
USMG	US Medical Graduate
PGY	Post-Graduate Year

Contents

SECTION ONE: INTRODUCTION

1. Making the Decision to Train in the US 3
   Vijayprasad Gopichandran, Mohanakrishnan G

SECTION TWO: TAKING THE EXAMS

2. The United States Medical Licensing Examinations (USMLE)—An Introduction 15
   Paari Murugan, Muralikrishna G
3. Acing the USMLE Step 1 32
   Paari Murugan
4. Acing the USMLE Step 2 CK (Clinical Knowledge) 41
   Paari Murugan
5. The USMLE Step 2 CS: How to Prepare 47
   Dhinager Nandagopal
6. The USMLE Step 2 CS: High Yield Notes 55
   Jayashree Sundararajan
7. Acing the USMLE Step 3 65
   Dhinager Nandagopal
8. The USMLE Step 3: High Yield Notes 69
   Muralikrishna G

SECTION THREE: ENTERING THE UNITED STATES— THE BOTTLENECKS

9. Tourist Visa (B1/B2) 77
   Dhinager Nandagopal
10. Student Visa (F1) 83
    Jayashree Sundararajan
11. Other Routes of Entering the United States 96
    Muralikrishna G

SECTION FOUR: ADDING WEIGHT TO YOUR APPLICATION

12. Research Before Residency 101
    Varun Agarwal
13. United States Clinical Experience (USCE) 107
    Muralikrishna G

SECTION FIVE: THE PROCESS OF GETTING INTO A US RESIDENCY

14. Choosing A Specialty 117
    Nirav Mamdani
15. J1 Vs H-1B—The Million Dollar Question 121
    Nirav Mamdani
16. The Nuts and Bolts of Residency Application 125
    Archana Bhaskaran, Muralikrishna G

SECTION SIX: CUSTOMIZING YOUR APPLICATION FOR YOUR SPECIALTY

17. Internal Medicine 147
    Vijayprasad Gopichandran, Nirav Mamdani
18. Pediatrics 156
    Chandrasekhar Yangalsetty
19. Psychiatry 160
    Aditi Malik
20. Family Practice 168
    Vandana Panda Goyle
21. Obstetrics and Gynecology 172
    Baraa Allaf M
22. Neurology 189
    Disha Uttam Shah
23. Surgery 196
    Pragatheeswar Thirunavukkarasu
24. Other Competitive Specialties 205
    Muralikrishna G

SECTION SEVEN: WHAT AFTER THE MATCH?

25. You Matched, Then What? 209
    Archana Bhaskaran

SECTION EIGHT: MISCELLANEOUS

26. Suggested Reading, Website Links, Official Links 215
    Muralikrishna G
27. Frequently Asked Questions (FAQs) 219
    Muralikrishna G
28. Program Director Speaks 226
    Jayashree Sundararajan
29. Sample Documents 228
    Muralikrishna G and Jayashree Sundararajan

    Index 257

Section One
Introduction

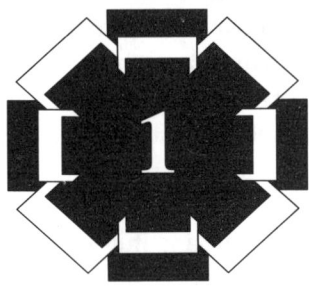

Making the Decision to Train in the US

Vijayprasad Gopichandran, Mohanakrishnan G

WHAT AFTER MEDICAL SCHOOL?

This is a major question facing all of us who pass out of our MBBS. It is a personal decision for each of us. For a few it is a part of a dream journey from high school to medical college and from there to the United States residency. For some of us it is a deep fascination and admiration of some senior colleague or teacher who has had his/her training in the US. But the largest group of us is that "fortunate" (or should we say unfortunate!!!) bunch which does not really know if we want to do a residency in the US or want to explore the option. It is not far off before the 'wily mistress' called US residency throws her willful trap on us! We definitely need some help to make the decision to go to the US for residency training. This chapter is written targeted at us, to help us make a well-informed decision.

After the struggle of the last few days drudging through the internship chores, at last the MBBS course is over. There is a lot of celebration and party! What next? There are several choices out there.

The first choice is that of entering into clinical practice. This is becoming less popular in current times. Some daring heroes and some with passion for primary care and practice of medicine at the grass roots level take up private practice in rural settings. The other option is to enter government service through the State Public Service Commission Exams and the Union Public Service Commission Exams. The takers of these government jobs later on opt for their postgraduate training with special privileges for their post in government service.

4 Acing the USMLE and the Match

Another popular option after medical school seems to be pursuing a postgraduate training in one of the premier institutes in India namely All India Institute of Medical Sciences, Postgraduate Institute of Medical Education and Research, JIPMER, etc. These institutions have their respective entrance exams. Preparation for these entrance exams is a challenge in its own respect. Then there is the All India Postgraduate Entrance Exam conducted annually for a fixed percentage of Postgraduate seats in all the teaching institutes in the country. This is another challenging exam with its own school of preparation and training. The State Entrance exams conducted by the directorate of medical education of each state allot postgraduate training positions to its own medical graduates.

The third and by far the most popular option seems to be going abroad for a postgraduate training. The United States, the United Kingdom, Canada, Australia, New Zealand and Singapore have enticing opportunities for medical training positions and employment. The two tables, Table 1.1 and Table 1.2 illustrate the fact that these developed countries have a large contingent of foreign doctors especially Indians in their health care workforce.

Table 1.1: Percentage of IMGs in the workforce in the four major developed countries

Country	Percentage of IMG in workforce	Percentage of IMG from developing countries
United States	25%	60%
United Kingdom	28%	75%
Canada	23%	43%
Australia	27%	40%

IMG – International Medical Graduate

Table 1.2: Percentage of Indians in the workforce in the four major developed countries

Country	Percentage of Indians in the workforce
United States	5%
United Kingdom	11%
Canada	2%
Australia	4%

India and the Indian subcontinent provide the largest number of doctors to the developed countries. The emigration factor for India (defined as the proportion of the Indian doctors who work in the developed countries as compared to the total doctors graduating from India) is the second highest among all countries in the developing world. It is reported that approximately 1200 Indian doctors leave for the US every year to take up residency training.

Thus it is a documented fact that there is a burgeoning trend of doctors going abroad to train. The scope of this chapter is to consider the option of going to the United States for training.

Popular Reasons why one wants to do a Residency in the US

1. The single most important reason why one would choose to do a residency in the United States is the idea that the training in the US is the best. Though "best" could be a very subjective term there are several popular explanations provided for it:
   i. US Residency is like a boot camp. It makes you work hard and thus brings out the best in you.
   ii. It imbibes in you work ethics and a healthy work culture.
   iii. It trains everybody rigorously and makes all rise to a particular standard
   iv. It teaches best evidence-based practices…
   v. US is the most happening place in the technological advances in medicine and thus it gives hands-on exposure to these advances.
2. Another important reason is the socioeconomic leap that is associated with working in the US. Bigger earnings and better lifestyle is any day a luring prospect that tempts one to take up the US training option. Not only is it lucrative if one emigrates to the US, even if one decides to return to India after a training, the pay package is significantly hefty given the US training and the experience.
3. Fancy specializations and superspecializations are thought to be more available and feasible in the US. It is oft-quoted: "In the US, if there is enterprise and commitment anything can be accomplished". For the Indian doctor whose thoughts are restricted and curbed by the system, this is a liberating option and often reason enough to choose to go to the US.
4. For many the negative psychology is the main reason for the US choice. Frustrations with the system of education and the methods of selection to enter a postgraduate training program in India leads to a negative feeling against training at home. Escaping from the restraints of the Indian system and reaching the American process which seems more regularized and merit-based is the reason why some choose an American residency training.
5. Another reason why you would think about USMLE over other options, especially if you have decided to undergo residency training abroad is the recent change in the medical education system in the United Kingdom. By and large, the Modernizing Medical Careers (MMC) and the Work Permit ruling have meant that the United Kingdom is no longer a viable option for a medical graduate from the Indian sub-continent.

6 Acing the USMLE and the Match

A detailed look at the option of the United Kingdom follows here since the US and the UK are the commonest routes available to medical students and graduates when it comes to going abroad.

UK: A CLOSED DOOR FOR IMGS?

Current trends and employment prospects

On 7 March, 2006 the Department of Health announced that from 3 April, 2006 IMGs—who are not UK or EEA nationals—wishing to work or train in the UK will need a work permit. To obtain a work permit an employer must show that a genuine vacancy exists, which cannot be filled by a doctor who is a UK or an EEA national. IMGs employment prospects will significantly worsen following the Department of Health announcement on 7 March, 2006. This is in addition to the on-going difficulties IMGs have reported in seeking employment.

Traditional route for PG medical training in UK for IMGs

General Medical Council registration is required before you can practise medicine in the UK. The first step is to gain 'limited registration' which will enable you to practise in the National Health Service (NHS) in supervised employment.
1. Evidence of English language skills (satisfactory IELTS scores).
2. Before you can be granted limited registration you must provide the GMC with evidence of your medical knowledge and skills (passes at Part 1 and Part 2 of the PLAB test).
3. Evidence of good standing from MCI.
4. Evidence that you have the offer of a suitable job.

Passing the IELTS

You have to obtain the following minimum scores in the Academic component: Overall 7, Speaking 7, Listening 6, Academic reading 6, Academic writing 6. This test is supposed to take a minimum of two weeks preparation. You may be able to obtain study material (books and tapes), and book for this exam via your local British Council centre.

Cracking the PLAB

To take the PLAB test you must have an acceptable primary medical qualification published by the World Health Organisation.

Making the Decision to Train in the US   7

The test is in two parts:

Part 1 is a written paper consisting of extended matching questions (EMQs) and single best answer (SBA) questions. The paper contains 200 questions and may contain photographic material. It lasts three hours. The proportion of SBA questions may vary from examination to examination but no more than 30% of the paper is composed of SBA questions. You can have an unlimited number of attempts but you must pass Part 1 within two years of the date of your IELTS certificate.

Recommended books for PLAB 1 include Oxford Handbook of Clinical Medicine (OHCM) and Oxford Handbook of Clinical Specialties (OHCS). This exam is supposed to be relatively easy to crack for standard Indian IMGs.

Part 2 is an Objective Structured Clinical Examination (OSCE). It takes the form of 14 clinical scenarios or 'stations', a rest station and a pilot station. Each station lasts five minutes. You must pass Part 2 within three years of passing Part 1. You can have four attempts at Part 2. If you fail at the fourth attempt you will have to retake IELTS (unless you are exempt) and both parts of the PLAB test.

Part 2 coaching centres in the UK include PLAB Master, PLAB tutor and PLAB trainer. Overall, an unpredictable exam requiring demonstration of clinical and communication skills. This exam is supposed to take a minimum of three weeks preparation.

You must be granted limited registration within three years of passing Part 2 of the test.

Recommended books for PLAB 1 include Oxford Handbook of Clinical Medicine (OHCM) and Oxford Handbook of Clinical Specialties (OHCS).

Clinical attachments

Doctors can undertake short periods of clinical attachment in the UK. As these are unpaid and involve observation only and not treatment of patients, doctors will still be able to take these posts while they are in the UK to take PLAB. Useful websites include drfoster.co.uk, specialistinfo.com, UK Deanery and the respective Royal College websites.

By and large, the UK has become a closed option after the introduction of the Modernizing Medical Careers (MMC) and the recent Work Permit ruling. Even in the old system, competitive specialties were hard to come by for foreign doctors and one had to find a new job every six months. Considering all these factors, one has to come to a decision about where one wants to ultimately train. With countries like Australia, Singapore, West Indies and some in the Middle

East offering lucrative jobs especially in their Areas of Need (AON), it is an option a number of medical graduates, especially with Postgraduate experience are now considering. The caveat here, being the lack of structured training and the lack of knowledge of how the degree obtained will be recognized in your home country.

While these are the common reasons why one decides to pursue residency training in the US, the decision buck does not stop here. There are several important factors to be considered before plunging into the sea called US residency!

Factors to be considered while making the decision:

1. *The United States Medical Licensing Exams or USMLE* is the first and often considered the rate-limiting step of this US residency endeavour. Twenty-four long hours of rigorous examination for certification (eight hours of USMLE Step 1 + eight hours of USMLE Step 2 CK + eight hours of USMLE Step 2 CS), seventeen more hours of exam for the licensing (nine hours on day one of USMLE Step 3 and eight hours on day two of USMLE Step 3)!!! The challenge faced by the Indian doctor in dealing with these exams is the fact that the Indian medical education system barring a few exceptions does not prepare the doctor to think laterally which is an essential aspect of these exams. Preparation for these exams requires a lot of "unlearning" and "relearning" of facts, concepts and ideas. Many times there is also a need to reorient one's thinking from the traditional Indian ways to the more American ways. This might mean a lot of hard work, efforts and struggle in the beginning.

2. *The Financial Investment* that is required for venturing into the process of entering an American residency is quite huge. The rough cost involved in taking the exams alone (approximate costs subject to changes) is Rupees one lakh and sixty three thousand as provided in Table 1.3. Added to this would be the cost of residency applications, document processing, and travel to the US to attend interviews, visa processing and finally the settling in expenses, which amount to a total of Rupees four lakh in addition. The cost break up is provided in Table 1.4. The fact that the cost involved in venturing into an Indian postgraduate training might not even be one tenth of this investment might be a factor to be considered before taking the big step. One argument which is often given is that the financial incentives that one gets after the training in the United States more than compensate for this initial investment.

3. *Career Objectives* have to be clearly defined before deciding to go to the US for residency training. What motivates one doctor is entirely different from what

Making the Decision to Train in the US

Table 1.3: Cost of taking the USMLE

S. No	Exam Name	Cost in USD	Cost in Indian Rupees (Approximate)
1	USMLE Step 1	845	39,000
2	USMLE Step 2 CK	860	40,000
3	USMLE Step 2 CS	1200	55,000
4	USMLE Step 3	635	29,000

Table 1.4: Miscellaneous expenses for the US residency route

S. No	Expense	Cost in USD	Cost in Indian Rupees (Approximate)
1	ERAS Token	75	3500
2	ERAS Application Fees (For fifty programs approximately)	790	36000
3	NRMP Fees	90	4000
4	NRMP Rank Order List fees (For 20 programs approximately)	150	7000
5	Document preparation	100	4600
6	Travel expenses to the US	1500	69000
7	Travel for interviews and stay in the US	2000	92000
8	Visa Processing (Variable for J1 and H1b)	2000	92000
9	Settling in the US	2000	92000

motivates another. There are doctors whose passion is working at the level of the masses. There are others whose dream is to be the authority with a niche of their own in an extremely super specialized field. For example, for that doctor who wants to work in a small village in Bihar for the betterment of health care delivery there, the US residency route seems a little too much in the plate. On the other hand for that aspiring fetal cardio-thoracic surgeon the US might be the best place to be trained.

4. *Feasibility of obtaining a residency of choice in the US* is a very important limiting factor in making the decision. If you were trying to pursue, say Neurosurgery or Orthopedic Surgery or such ultra-competitive specialties in the US, it would help to sit down and make an honest appraisal of what chances you actually have of getting into such a specialty in the United States. Some specialties are extremely difficult to get into. Some are easier for International Medical Graduates (IMGs). This depends on the relative competitiveness of each of these specialties. Some specialties might be particularly popular among the American graduates in which case IMGs might not be welcome into those specialties. Table 1.5 tabulates the percentage of international

medical graduates accepted into the residency training programs in various specialties in the US (statistics from the year 2004).

Table 1.5: Percentage of International Medical Graduates accepted into the various specialties in a year (statistics of the year 2004).

S. No	Specialty	Percentage of residents that are IMGs
1	Family Medicine	38.1%
2	**Internal Medicine**	**50.8%**
3	Neurology	38.1%
4	Pathology	42.5%
5	Surgery	21.8%
6	Emergency Medicine	5.9%
7	Obstetrics and Gynecology	23.3%
8	Ophthalmology	6.9%
9	Otolaryngology	2.4%
10	Pediatrics	31.9%
11	Psychiatry	39.7%
12	Radiology	8.3%

5. *The Big Divide:* The divide is between doing a specialty of choice and getting world-class training. If one decides to go to the US for residency training there might have to be some compromise on the specialty of choice and the place where one wants to train in the US. On the other hand, there are other viable alternative options such as remaining in India, going to the UK or Australia, where the chances of getting a specialty of choice might be much easier. The bridge over this major divide is the long term objectives and career goals of the individual and it is a difficult personalized decision.

The Ultimate decision making process

So far the chapter has targeted on bringing into focus the options after medical school, the reasons why one might find the US residency option interesting and the various important factors to be considered before making the choice. An important factor to be considered is one of financial risk, where you may end up spending a few lakhs of rupees only to find out that the US Consulate will not grant you a visa to take the USMLE Step 2 CS exam. Ultimately, the decision is a very personal one and it rests solely on the individual. This chapter is not written to encourage one to enter into a US residency. It is written to guide the thinking process of those who have the idea in their mind. After reading this chapter one might be encouraged to pursue the US residency path or might be dissuaded from it. Both are welcome outcomes of this chapter. It is mainly written as a primer to the whole process of the US residency. The chapter concludes wishing all its readers a meaningful decision, making process.

REFERENCES

1. http://www.ama-assn.org/vapp/freida/spcindx/0,,TR,00.html
2. http://www.ecfmg.org/
3. Fitzhugh Mullan. The Metrics of the Physician Brain Drain. New Engl J Med. 2005; 353: 1810-1818.
4. Fitzhugh Mullan. Doctors for the World - Indian Physician emigration. Health Affairs. 2006; 25(2): 380-393. http://content.healthaffairs.org/cgi/content/full/25/2/380

Section Two
Taking the Exams

The United States Medical Licensing Examinations (USMLE) — An Introduction

Paari Murugan, Muralikrishna G

The United States Medical Licensing Examination™ (USMLE™) is a three-step examination for medical licensure in the United States and is sponsored by the Federation of State Medical Boards (FSMB) and the National Board of Medical Examiners® (NBME®).

The Composite Committee, appointed by the FSMB and NBME, establishes rules for the USMLE program. Membership includes representatives from the FSMB, NBME, Educational Commission for Foreign Medical Graduates (ECFMG®), and the American public.

In the United States and its territories ("United States" or "US"), the individual medical licensing authorities ("State Medical Boards") of the various jurisdictions grant a license to practise medicine. Each medical licensing authority sets its own rules and regulations and requires passing an examination that demonstrates qualification for licensure. Results of the USMLE are reported to these authorities for use in granting the initial license to practise medicine. The USMLE provides them with a common evaluation system for applicants for medical licensure.

The USMLE assesses a physician's ability to apply knowledge, concepts, and principles, and to demonstrate fundamental patient-centred skills that are important in health and disease and that constitute the basis of safe and effective patient care. Each of the three Steps complements the others; no Step can stand alone in the assessment of readiness for medical licensure. Because individual medical licensing authorities make decisions regarding use of USMLE results, you should contact the jurisdiction where you intend to apply for licensure to obtain complete information. Also, the FSMB can provide general information on medical licensure.

16　Acing the USMLE and the Match

USMLE MISSION STATEMENT

The United States Medical Licensing Examination (USMLE) program supports medical licensing authorities in the United States through its leadership in the development, delivery, and continual improvement of high quality assessments across the continuum of physicians' preparation for practise.

Goals:

To provide to licensing authorities meaningful information from assessments of physician characteristics—including medical knowledge, skills, values, and attitudes—that are important to the provision of safe and effective patient care.

To engage medical educators and their institutions, licensing authority members, and practicing clinicians in the design and development of these assessments.

To assure fairness and equity to physicians through the highest professional testing standards.

To continue to develop and improve assessments for licensure with the intent of assessing physicians more accurately and comprehensively.

THE THREE STEPS OF THE USMLE

Step 1 assesses whether you understand and can apply important concepts of the sciences basic to the practise of medicine, with special emphasis on principles and mechanisms underlying health, disease, and modes of therapy. Step 1 ensures mastery of not only the sciences that provide a foundation for the safe and competent practice of medicine in the present, but also the scientific principles required for maintenance of competence through lifelong learning.

Step 2 assesses whether you can apply medical knowledge, skills, and understanding of clinical sciences essential for the provision of patient care under supervision and includes emphasis on health promotion and disease prevention. Step 2 ensures that due attention is devoted to principles of clinical sciences and basic patient-centred skills that provide the foundation for the safe and competent practise of medicine.

Step 3 assesses whether you can apply medical knowledge and understanding of biomedical and clinical sciences essential for the unsupervised practise of medicine, with emphasis on patient management in ambulatory settings. Step 3 provides a final assessment of physicians assuming independent responsibility for delivering general medical care.

The permutations and combinations of the number of questions available in the USMLE question pool from which the questions are picked make it a unique

The USMLE—An Introduction

experience for each and every test-taker. Although each experience is vastly different, it is possible to derive invaluable lessons from the experiences of others that can help scores of new generation of IMG- USMLE test-takers to compete more successfully.

Breaking up the discussion into a few meaningful headers should serve the purpose better so as to clearly define all possible doubts and ambiguities and put forth what actually is to be done. We shall try and answer as much as possible through the following:
1. When should the exams be taken?
2. In what order should they be taken?
3. How do I apply for and schedule the exam?
4. How do I prepare for the USMLE?
5. How long should the preparation time be?
6. Am I ready to start studying? Do I need a study partner?
7. Am I ready to take the exam?
8. Pre-exam day strategies
9. Exam day strategies
10. Getting the score!
11. I got my score, then what?

General chronological time-frame for any USMLE exam:
1. Get all background information about the exam from the official USMLE website, USMLE forums, friends, college seniors.
2. Get the necessary study materials ready and put up a tentative time-table.
3. Apply for and schedule the exam.
4. Stick to the time-table and prepare for the exam.
5. Begin solving MCQs along with your core preparatory materials.
6. Ask yourself: Am I ready to take the exam.
7. Take the exam.
8. Get your score...Yahoo!

1. WHEN SHOULD THE EXAMS BE TAKEN?

The decision about when to take the exam is very closely related to when the decision is made by the individual to plunge into the path to residency in the United States.

The sooner the decision is made about the US, the better. Ideally this would be around the time you are trudging through the fag end of second year. Understandably it is difficult making a definitive career plan that early. Though very few who went through the process have ever done so, we shall initially discuss the ideal and then look at other options. The pros and cons of destination USA is discussed in detail elsewhere in this book and here it will suffice to say just this—make sure you are at least mentally oriented for all the Indian PG entrances as well. Blind faith in the US Consulate is akin to dozing off with a ticking time bomb under the pillow! Putting up a tentative schedule at the end of second year and planning on taking Step 1 sometime in third year will be on the dot as it gives you enough time in internship to maneuver around for the Indian exams as well. Also, one will be relatively fresh from the basic sciences, which Step 1 is all about. On the other hand, it may be better to go for the Step 1 after a fuller grasp of the clinics, since it is much easier to correlate and work through the conceptual questions that will be raised in the test. Indeed confusing and doesn't look like it helps much talking both ways but it all depends on how well you have been going about trying to master the basic sciences as a fledgling medico. If you have been the happy-go-lucky kind and done nothing much but basked in pseudo glory of the "Man I'm a medico! Ain't that cool!" feeling, maybe you ought to wait a bit and go for plan B. So, coming back to the ideal, take Step 1 sometime in third year, which is the coolest of the MBBS days, and plan Step 2 so that you can take it after one of the not-so-tough rotations in internship.

This way you will be ready to fly right away after internship and make use of the time cushion till the interviews at the end of the year to look around for observerships. In the meantime Step 2 CS and Step 3 can be handled with comfort. This is also of major importance since you do find more space to study for and squeeze in the Indian exams if forced to wait, owing to visa refusals, till the next year.

So then, what are the other seemingly less than ideal options?

If not totally convinced about your grasp of the basic sciences or had never given a thought about all this till after final MBBS, never fear, it still can be done without waiting an extra year if you break just a little more sweat. Try and take at least Step 1 during or just after internship. Doing both requires huge commitment and a good slice of luck too, in the sense the units with which you are posted should be on the cooler side. Anyhow it won't make much difference if you take the second exam a few months after graduating, other than rob you of an AIIMS/PGI entrance alongside. It is common knowledge that the MLE preparation is never going to be enough to get you through into the higher rank lists of these mundane factual exams, though without doubt, conceptwise the MLE prep will keep you well ahead of the others. After Step 2, work on the visa interviews while hitting the Indian MCQ books. Preparation for Step 2 CS can well be done after the visa is confirmed.

One other option of course is, if the time-frame is not a bother or if the internship had been too hectic, to start after graduation, sit with the books for a year and take Step 1, Step 2 plus the Indian exams and go for the next match. Two birds in one stone and its no longer life or death. There's always motherland PG to lean back on and this in a way may offer some assistance in getting a visa.

Some universities are said to prefer candidates who have not been "wasting" any time, but it does not seem to matter much at most places.

2. IN WHAT ORDER SHOULD THEY BE TAKEN?

The best advice is to take it as they come... 1, 2 and then CS. The one condition where the consideration can be otherwise is, if you have financial difficulties. In that case, apply for Step 2 CS (CS fee is refundable) and try getting the visa. If that works out, take it first (in case the visa is not a multiple entry type) and then plan for Steps 1 and 2 after you come back. Again it's not assured that you will get a visa for the interviews if you have not got the multiple entry visa first time around. The risk of not getting the visa the second time especially after coming back is much lower though. This issue is discussed elsewhere in the book. It is beyond the scope of this section to discuss other "methods" of working out the visa part.

It's quite ill-advised as a first time USMLE taker to change the order of Steps 1 and 2. Step 1 for one thing is easier and helps in getting oriented towards tackling these exams. Moreover, preparing for the first helps a long way in understanding concepts, which are vital for tackling Step 2. There is that argument which floats around saying its easier taking Step 2 first after internship or final year for that matter as one is fresh from the clinics. Always remember—the American clinics are way different from ours and the intricacies of the Step 2 exam are not quite reflected in Indian teaching and in the type of "exam-based" cases, which we get to see here.

3. HOW DO I APPLY FOR AND SCHEDULE THE EXAM?

If you are a Medical Student

To be eligible for **Step 1, Step 2 CK, and Step 2 CS**, you must be officially enrolled in a medical school located outside the United States and Canada that is listed in the *International Medical Education Directory (IMED)* of the Foundation for Advancement of International Medical Education and Research (FAIMER), both at the time that you apply and at the time you take the exam. In addition, the "Graduation Years" in *IMED* for your medical school must be listed as "Current" at the time you apply and at the time you take the exam. Your Medical

School Dean, Vice Dean, or Registrar must certify your current enrollment status on the application. This certification must be **current**; the official must have signed the application within **four months** of its receipt by ECFMG. As soon as you graduate and receive your medical diploma, you must send two photocopies of your medical diploma and one full-face color photograph to ECFMG (see *Provision of Credentials and Translations*). The photograph that you send must be current; it must have been taken within six months of the date that you send it. A photocopy of a photograph is not acceptable.

In addition to being currently enrolled as described above, to be eligible for Step 1, Step 2 CK, and Step 2 CS, you must have completed at least two years of medical school. This eligibility requirement means that you must have completed the basic medical science component of the medical school curriculum by the beginning of your eligibility period.

Although you may apply for and take the examinations after completing the basic medical science component of your medical school curriculum, you should consider the following recommendations before applying for Step 2 CK and Step 2 CS. Before taking Step 2 CK and Step 2 CS, it is recommended that you complete your core clinical clerkships, including actual patient contact.

ECFMG reserves the right to reverify with the medical schools the eligibility of medical school students who are registered for an exam. If ECFMG requests reverification of your student status with your medical school, ECFMG will release your score report only after reverification of your status has been received by ECFMG.

If you have already graduated from Medical College

To be eligible for Step 1, Step 2 CK, and Step 2 CS, you must be a graduate of a medical school located outside the United States and Canada that is listed in the *International Medical Education Directory (IMED)* of the Foundation for Advancement of International Medical Education and Research (FAIMER). Your graduation year must be included in the medical school's *IMED* listing. You must have had at least four credit years (academic years for which credit has been given toward completion of the medical curriculum) in attendance at a medical school that is listed in *IMED*. The signature of the official who certifies your status as a graduate on the application must be **current**; the official must have signed the application within **four months** of its receipt by ECFMG.

You must also submit two photocopies of your medical diploma at the time of application if you have not sent the diploma to ECFMG previously. One full-face color photograph must accompany the copies of your diploma. The photograph that you send must be **current**; it must have been taken within six months of the date that you send your application. A photocopy of a photograph is not acceptable. If your medical diploma has not yet been issued, you must submit with the application a current color photograph and a letter signed by your Medical School Dean, Vice Dean, or Registrar that confirms you graduated from medical school, have met all requirements to receive your medical diploma, and states the date (month and year) that your medical diploma will be issued. You must then send the photocopies of your medical diploma to ECFMG as soon as your diploma is issued. You must also complete and submit with your medical diploma or letter from your medical school the *ECFMG Medical Education Credentials Submission Form* (Form 344) and *Medical School Release Request* (Form 345).

The name on your medical diploma and/or letter from your medical school must match **exactly** the name in your ECFMG record. If the names do not match **exactly**, you must submit legal documentation that **verifies** the name on your medical diploma and/or letter from your medical school is (or was) your name.

Applying for Examination

You can apply **online** using ECFMG's Interactive Web Application (IWA) or download a paper application from this website and send the completed application to ECFMG.

You may not register using a letter, postcard, or e-mail message. All photographs, signatures, and seals/stamps on the application must be original. You cannot register by faxing your application or sending photocopies of the application to ECFMG.

Detailed instructions accompany both the online and paper applications. Follow the instructions carefully and answer all questions completely. You should review the instructions **before** you begin working on the application. Some of the necessary items require advance planning. These items include photographs, official signatures, and additional documentation, such as copies of your medical diploma if you are a medical school graduate. If your application is not complete, it will be rejected.

ECFMG will notify you when your application is received. If you provide an e-mail address when you apply, ECFMG will send this notification by e-mail. If you do not provide an e-mail address, ECFMG will send this notification by postal mail. You can check the status of your exam application online using OASIS.

ECFMG will process your application and payment and determine your eligibility to take the exam(s) you requested. Once your application has been processed, ECFMG will notify you of the outcome of your application. For eligible applicants, ECFMG will also send important information about scheduling and taking the exams.

Important note: Application and other requests for services will not be processed if it is determined that doing so would be violative of any applicable federal laws or regulations.

Applying Online

Access IWA on this website. ECFMG processes online applications typically within ten business days of receipt of the complete application.

Students

Medical school students who use IWA must print a Certification Statement (Form 183) after completing the online portion of the application and return the completed Form 183 to ECFMG. Students must complete and submit Form 183 for **each** online application.

Form 183 must be completed by the student and certified by an appropriate official of the student's medical school. This certification must be **current**; the official must have signed the form within four months of its receipt by ECFMG.

Any additional documentation that is required at the time of application must be submitted with Form 183. The only items that should not be submitted with Form 183 are requests and supporting documentation for test accommodations.

Online applications from students are not considered complete until ECFMG receives the completed Form 183 accompanied by any other required documents.

You can access Form 183 from IWA after completing the online portion of the application.

Graduates

Effective August 31, 2005, the online application process has been simplified for medical school graduates. Graduates who apply online on/after August 31, 2005 must print a *Certification of Identification Form* (Form 186) after completing the online portion of the application and return the completed Form 186 to ECFMG. Once accepted by ECFMG, this form remains valid for online applications received during the following five-year period, and subsequent applications during this period can be completed entirely online.

Form 186 must be completed by the graduate and certified by an appropriate official. This certification must be current; the official must have signed the form within four months of its receipt by ECFMG.

The USMLE—An Introduction 23

Any additional documentation that is required at the time of application, including Form 186, must be accompanied by a completed *IWA Document Submission Form* (Form 187) to ensure that it is matched with the online portion of the application.

Online applications from graduates are not considered complete until the completed Form 186 (if required) and any other required documents are received at ECFMG. All required documents must be sent in one envelope, accompanied by Form 187.

Submitting a paper application

Download paper application materials from the Publications page of this website or request a photocopy from ECFMG. Processing time for paper applications is approximately four weeks.

For both students and graduates, each paper application must be certified by an appropriate official. This certification must be current; the official must have signed the form within four months of its receipt by ECFMG.

Any additional documentation that is required at the time of application must be submitted with the application.

WHEN TO APPLY

Step 1, Step 2 CK, and Step 2 CS are offered regularly throughout the year; however, there may be occasional, brief periods when all test centers are closed or the exam is not available. There is no deadline for submitting your exam application. However, the application materials specify a date after which you cannot use them and must use the next year's application materials. You should check for this date before you apply. In planning the timing of your application, refer to *Eligibility Periods* on the ECFMG website for information on how eligibility periods are assigned. You should also consider deadlines imposed by the National Resident Matching Program (NRMP) and Graduate Medical Education (GME) programs. You should be aware that demand for test dates/centers at certain times during the year may exceed the number of testing spaces available.

Fees

You must pay all applicable fees at the time of application. If you apply for more than one exam at the same time, you must pay applicable fees for **all** exams at the time of application. **If you do not pay all fees, your application will be rejected.** If your application is rejected, any payment received with that

24 Acing the USMLE and the Match

application will be credited to your ECFMG financial account.

For Step 1 or Step 2 CK, the total fee consists of the examination fee plus the appropriate international test delivery surcharge, if applicable.

Examination Fee. The examination fee for 2006 eligibility periods was $ 695 for each exam. All applicants must pay the examination fee.

International Test Delivery Surcharge

If you choose a testing region other than the United States/Canada, you must also pay the international test delivery surcharge for the international testing region that you choose. These surcharges represent the additional cost of offering Step 1 and Step 2 CK by computer outside the United States and Canada. If you choose to take the exam in the United States or Canada, you do not need to pay a surcharge. For information on Step 1/Step 2 CK testing regions, refer to *Testing Locations* on the ECFMG website.

For Step 2 CS, the fee for 2006 applications was $ 1,200.

4. HOW DO I PREPARE FOR THE USMLE?

- Stick to one set of study materials
- Kaplan notes for each of the Steps are sufficient for most subjects and can take your percentile scores into the low 90s. (vide chapters 3 and 4 for a detailed discussion)
- Questions, questions and more questions.... solving more and more questions is the key to tackling the USMLE. There are umpteen number of question banks available for the USMLE, but the ones most commonly used and the ones we would like to recommend and that are closest to the real exam are Kaplan Q bank and Q book for USMLE Step 1, USMLE World MCQs for USMLE Step 2, USMLE World CCS for Step 3.
- NBME (National Board of Medical Examiners) offers online simulated testing just like the real exam prior to the exam and offers a chance to assess whether you are ready for the real exam or not.
- Another useful study strategy is to finish the Kaplan notes for each individual subject and to immediately do questions from the subjectwise Kaplan Q bank.
- Once you have finished all the Kaplan notes or all the subjects with the corresponding questions from Kaplan Q bank, you can revise the Kaplan notes and start doing the Kaplan Q book.

5. HOW LONG SHOULD THE PREPARATION TIME BE?

This is by far the quintessential question on the topic. That it depends on individual abilities is probably a redundant statement. Nevertheless, one needs to have a general idea so as to make it easier to gauge and set up an indigenous timetable.

The oft-repeated lines you see on Internet links goes like this:

Two months for Step 1, two weeks for Step 2 and two days for Step 3.

This idea is a good joke at best.

The Americans who always take the steps before the course is over have put it up. It's a pretty tight schedule for them and they can't financially and/or otherwise for various reasons afford to wait longer, plus the scores are less important to them than passing the test.

Since the American universities have no way of assessing IMGs before the interviews unless you are from AIIMS or have done an observership in the US, whatever said and done you have to go for maximum. Agreed, once you get the interview calls they may not be of much importance.

Three to four months will be the ideal average prep time for Step 1. Two to three months would suffice for Step 2.

How long to prepare and what to use as study materials is highly variable and we would not like to give hard and fast rules regarding this. It is imperative to stress that the USMLE does not test rote learning like the Indian exams and hence concept-oriented learning would help a lot more whatever study materials you use.

This time period is sufficient when you have completed MBBS and have all day to spare. If not, a month or two more to be on the safer side.

On a three-month schedule 9-11 hrs a day of study should be perfect. Make it 7-9 if you are the whiz-kid kind who has enviable powers of concentration/perseverance. When doing the preparation in between course, adjust your timings based on the above.

The unique thing about the USMLE exams is that you can set your own D-Day. As Indian students, never in our academic lives have we had that kind of luxury. This lulls one into putting the test off till there is enough "confidence". Believe me, beyond a particular point that is just a wishful thought.

The trick here is to take the exam sooner than later, adding an extra month may be very tempting but is never going to help if you are planning on going through the notes just that one last time. The tendency to forget the initial lessons as time creeps by is a well-known caveat and it's pretty tough trying to juggle more than two subjects at a time.

26 Acing the USMLE and the Match

For the USMLE it's the cumulative knowledge that matters. Memorizing notes is as pathetic an idea as it can get and is of absolutely no help.

Always remember, what you study is much more important than how long you study.

6. AM I READY TO START STUDYING? DO I NEED A STUDY PARTNER?

A short checklist before you start studying:
- Kaplan notes
- Kaplan Q bank
- Kaplan Q book
- Applying for and scheduling the exam
- Computer with Internet access (to connect with another USMLE taker)
- Credit card (need not be yours!)
- A study partner (Real or virtual!)

The USMLE forums (links to which are given at the end of book) are a very good source of information and to find friends who are preparing for the exam. A study partner can be very useful while preparing for the USMLE, especially when you are doing questions considering the fact that you and your study partner will have different areas of strength and weakness in various subjects. The USMLE forums are a good place to find study partners wherever in the world you are. Online study partners are also quite common and USMLE Yahoo groups have become good portals to form an online study group which are a very good place to discuss what to use, what to study and what questions to do. Whether you get a study partner, get a computer with Internet access and a credit card that you can use online to make payments. Note that the credit card need not necessarily be yours!

7. AM I READY TO TAKE THE EXAM?

For all the three USMLE Steps, once the Kaplan notes, Kaplan Q book and Q bank are done, the question is when to take the exam. There are three methods by which you can assess if you are ready.... NBME online testing, Kaplan simulated CD and the CD of 150 questions sent by USMLE.

A score of 70-80% on the simulated CD and 85-95% on the USMLE CD should be a comfortable score for you to schedule your exam in a month with revision especially the Kaplan notes supplemented with First Aid for each of the Steps. The NBME scores carrelate well with the actual USMLE scores with a variation of just one or two points.

8. PRE-EXAM DAY STRATEGIES

As crucial as your study preparation is the way you tune yourself up both physically and mentally for the exam. These exams are among the most exhausting and demanding ones on the planet. You need as much as possible to keep your wits razor sharp right from the word go till the last block of the day. This is almost like telling a marathon runner to run the same distance just after he's crossed the finish line! Impossible though it may seem, make sure you are in a position to put in your best effort. Keep to a fixed sleep pattern for at least the last two weeks leading into the exam and make sure the exam hours are your regular waking hours. Try and avoid taking afternoon naps. This really may not matter, as on exam day the adrenaline will be gushing so hard that an afternoon siesta will be the last thing on your mind! But it's wise to tune up the right way.

Prometric offers a practice test at their premises. This is not cost effective and is totally unnecessary. The same questions that are in the USMLE trial CD will be repeated. This you must do at home on the day before the exams. The exam itself is comparable but a bit tougher than the practice CD questions.

Be sure to get the tutorial clear so that you save on the exam and get more time for the breaks.

Get the books out of the way at least by dinner, preferably earlier. Try and be relaxed.

These exams are just not life or death. No exam ever is. Here you have the added advantage of taking it again, if you miss it for some reason. Far fetched though it may seem, it is possible. Take a very light non-oily dinner and get the stuff ready for the next day. Make sure of the orange card and the personal ID.

Food is not provided, so pack your things. A flask with steaming fresh coffee is a must. If you are by chance not a coffee drinker, take a caffeine substitute like a cola drink. Get some light eats like biscuits/cake and maybe some fruits. Water is provided at Prometric.

An 8-hour good night's sleep is so very vital for the next day. The exam almost equally tests your stamina as your knowledge. Keep a look out for non-hangover sedative pills as alternatives if you are the anxious kind.

9. EXAM DAY STRATEGIES

The test starts at nine. Be at the center at around eight thirty. Prometric conducts tests for lots of other specialties too and usually the GRE takers will be milling around. USMLE people will be called first. Get the locker key, put your things in and inform the proctor. Be as relaxed as you can. The hard work done will definitely pay dividends. A digital photo will be taken and the orange card confidential number will be torn and given to you along with a marker pen and a laminated sheet for rough work. Leave all other things in the locker and switch off the mobile.

In your cubicle, which is a bit like the Sify net center cubicles but with a little more privacy you will find earplugs, which may come in handy when the GRE guys start typing for the next four hours. In the afternoon you will be alone with the one or two other USMLE takers and left in peace. Reduce the screen brightness to a minimum to protect your eyes. Skip the tutorial and go straight to the test.

Take a break after every block. Step 1 has 7 and Step 2, 8. The total time is 8 and 9 hours respectively with 1 having 50 and 2, 46 questions in a block. Never make the mistake of doing two blocks continuously unless of course there is a break time crunch which is unlikely. Concentration will be in tatters towards the end of the second block if two blocks are taken continuously. Make sure the break screen is on when coming out every time.

Take the toilet break, splash your face with some cool water and every alternate block gets the caffeine/snacks in to keep the batteries running. Step out and have a walk if you feel like it but don't keep a break on for more than five to six minutes.

Don't linger on questions—the problem here is, some or rather most of the questions will be a mile long. It is not prudent to sit through and carefully read every line. Train yourself to scan quickly for clues. Many a time these questions will have the actual query as the last line. Always look for this eventuality first.

After you get the gist, work out the answer before looking at the choices. This way you don't fall for the problem of plenty. The first hit is almost always the best hit. If the answer is elusive, go for the elimination method. When nothing works, take a guess and move on.

There are times when you will be almost sure but not quite. Mark for later review and do not be hasty. These are the ones which fetch you valuable points.

It is also advisable to mark the unnaturally long ones right when you come across them instead of slaving through some jargon and finally realizing you have absolutely no clue. Indeed saves a lot of time especially on Step 2 where time is critical unlike Step 1, which is totally cool on the clock.

Complete the block and tend to all the unfinished business. Always do a revision if time permits. A new idea may strike, as you look at the question in an entirely different perspective. This is not meant for the ambiguous ones where as already said, the first hit is the best hit. Rather this helps weeding out the so-called "silly" mistakes.

The USMLE—An Introduction

Never leave a question unanswered for there are no negative marks. You cannot come back to a block once it's over.

The last few blocks are always the toughest. You will feel as exhausted as you have ever felt in your life. Don't give up—cling on, think of the question at hand and keep the concentration going. You are not going to let two hours undo the good work put in all these days.

If you are in time there is a feedback block at the end, which is optional. Get the receipt from the Prometric staff and get out—party all night, you deserved it… and forget about the exam however it may have been, you have done your best.

10. GETTING THE SCORE!

Your score is reported in about four weeks. Once your result is available, ECFMG will mail it to your ECFMG address of record. Results for Step 1/Step 2 CK are typically available in time to mail your report within three to four weeks after your test date. Results for Step 2 CS are typically available within eight weeks of your test date. However, delays are possible for various reasons. In selecting your test date and inquiring about results, you should allow at least eight weeks after your test date to receive your score report. You can check the status of your score report online using OASIS. To avoid misinterpretation and to protect the privacy of examinees, ECFMG will not provide scores or pass/fail outcomes by telephone, fax, or e-mail to anyone, including examinees.

Please note that the reporting of scores may be delayed if additional data and/or analyses are required to assure the validity of the test scores. Additionally, ECFMG reserves the right to reverify with the medical schools the eligibility of medical school students who are registered for examination. If ECFMG requests reverification of your student status with your medical school, ECFMG will release your score report only after reverification of your status has been received by ECFMG.

Step 1 / Step 2 CK

Score reports for Step 1 and Step 2 CK include a pass/fail designation, numerical scores, and graphical performance profiles, which summarize areas of strength and weakness to aid in self-assessment. These profiles are developed as assessment tools for the benefit of examinees only and are not reported or verified to third parties.

Except as otherwise specified below, to receive a score for Step 1/Step 2 CK, you must begin every block of the test. If you do not begin every block, no final results are reported, and the "incomplete examination" attempt appears on your USMLE transcript.

If your examination is incomplete, you may request that a score be calculated and reported, with all missed test items scored as incorrect. This score is likely to be lower than the score you would have achieved had you completed all sections of the examination. If you decide to request calculation and reporting of your score, the score will appear on your USMLE transcript as though it were complete. It will remain the permanent score for the examination administration. If your exam is incomplete, you will be notified in writing by NBME. You will have forty-five days from the date of this notification to request the exam to be scored as described above.

Step 2 CS

Performance on Step 2 CS is reported as pass or fail, with no numerical score. Examinees who fail receive graphical performance profiles, which reflect the relative strengths and weaknesses of the examinee's performance. These profiles are developed as assessment tools for the benefit of examinees only and are not reported or verified to third parties.

For Step 2 CS, if you do not begin every case, your performance may be assessed on those cases completed. If this assessment would result in a passing outcome no matter how poorly you may have performed on the missed case(s), then a "pass" will be reported. If this assessment would result in a failing outcome no matter how good your performance on the missed case(s), then a "fail" will be reported. Otherwise, the attempt may be recorded as an "incomplete examination."

11. I GOT MY SCORE, THEN WHAT?

The passing score is 75/ 182.

If you scored less than that and failed, it is a big blow or what. It is high time you rethought your decision and refocused on what went wrong in the preparation. The only good point is that you can retake the exam and get a better score on the exam.

Any score of 75-80 significantly reduces your chance of getting into a competitive specialty or competitive program but all is not lost. You can still work hard on the other steps and other parts of your application to make yourself a competitive candidate.

A score of 80-90 is good, but not great. The same issues apply and it would help to work harder on the other Steps or come to the realization of compromising on the specialty you want to go into or the kind of program you can get into.

A score in the 90s, especially the high nineties is just about perfect.

The ideal score is the 99 as the two digit score and high 260s or low 270s as the three digit score. This with a complete, all-round application gives you the best shot of competing for the competitive specialties and the competitive programs.

The USMLE is ultimately a test of the cumulative knowledge acquired through the years.

Most of us get that ability to conceptually analyze medical knowledge when we reach the fag end of the course and end up having some regrets as to how better it could have been planned in the initial days.

If you have the luxury of time, the post MBBS one year is a golden period, almost god sent for reliving the previously unexplored wonders of Medicine. Except for a few exceptional students, most of us, we believe, sat through our undergraduate days without much enthusiasm, be it due to uncharismatic teachers, lack of adequate personal will or a combination of both. This one year will help you get back most of what had been lost and maybe something even more as you are now in the perfect position to integrate and visualize the spellbinding complexities of the medical sciences.

Therein lies the beauty of the USMLE tests. They let you do exactly that, being least bothered about factual knowledge.

REFERENCES

http://www.acfmg.org/2007if/ifexam.html
http://www.usmle.org/bulletin/2007/toc.htm

Acing the USMLE Step 1

Paari Murugan

1. INTRODUCTION

Step 1 assesses whether you understand and can apply important concepts of the sciences basic to the practise of medicine, with special emphasis on principles and mechanisms underlying health, disease, and modes of therapy. Step 1 ensures mastery of not only the sciences that provide a foundation for the safe and competent practise of medicine in the present, but also the scientific principles required for maintenance of competence through lifelong learning. In general, Step 1 is more factual than Step 2 but the concept base required is a clear must.

2. WHAT ARE THE SUBJECTS TESTED?

The syllabus is drawn out in detail on the USMLE website but the primary subjects as we know are the following seven.
- Anatomy
- Physiology
- Biochemistry
- Microbiology
- Pharmacology
- Behavioral science
- Pathology

Other subjects that are commonly tested, but missed while preparing are Immunology, Genetics, Cell Biology, Molecular Biology, Acid-base balance, Nutrition, Biostatistics and HIV-AIDS.

3. WHAT STUDY MATERIALS TO USE?

Use the well known Kaplan notes as the core study material, though they are inadequate, to say the least, if you are going for a 95 plus percentile.

One day's test is always different from the other and since the questions are randomly generated, it is impossible to make a prediction on which subject your exam will lean towards.

Nevertheless, from experience and hearsay, you will hear that the exam will either be a Patho-Physiology based exam or Pharmacology based one with a good number of Pathology questions thrown in. An even mix of these is to be expected more often than not.

A crucial aspect of the exam that has to be underlined in bold is the role of Behavioral Science. Whatever is the nature of that particular day's test you can be 100% sure that the number of BS questions will be constant and will comprise up to 20-25% of the test. We will discuss in detail the same after sifting through a few general issues.

Start with Kaplan notes. Without doubt it's the best foundation from where you can build on. It gives you a drill of the core basics like no other book can.

The simplified text is so easy to understand and can be reviewed in such a short span that you are left wondering at the struggle you underwent during the preclinical years, poring through endless volumes of textbooks.

Split time so that you can give it one good reading plus an adequate revision. Squeezing in a complete second rapid revision at the end might give that extra bit of confidence going into the exam. Although, on exam day, confidence plays a vital role, I have to concede, the second revision probably is not a must.

What is a definite must is the amount of MCQs that have to be done.

Most of the knowledge required for the exams will be MCQ derived. There is never a limit—the more you do the better. Always go for the books which give detailed answer discussions. Go for MCQs as early in your preparation as you can. Give them equal, if not more, importance to the amount of notes being read.

The multifold advantages are:
1. There is exposure to a wider range of stuff in a short while and if you make sure to read through the discussion part carefully, the feeling of having learnt a lot in a limited period of time is undeniable. Not just a feeling, it's a fact. Poring through volumes of text and at the end of the day looking back at the number of pages may give you that sense of "accomplishment" but practically speaking, it pales in comparison to the sheer effectiveness of MCQ based reading.

2. MCQs are fun and interesting to do; they help give you refreshing breaks between text readings.
3. Worth its weight in gold is the time tested method of back reading where you do MCQs and go back to reading relevant material for all the choices given.

The best way to do these MCQs is to work out answers for a small set of questions, say around ten at a time and then go through the discussion part.

Though sitting with MCQs is fun, its hardwork going through the answers; but that's what ultimately pays. If you do a bulk of questions and then try to read the explanations there is always the risk of getting exhausted. Doing it on one-to-one basis is also a bit tiring.

During the last few days of the preparation get into the actual exam mode by doing 50 question blocks at a time, gradually getting the feel of the timed test.

It is not necessary to sit through a whole day and try simulating the actual exam. It doesn't really help and moreover whoever wants to undergo that kind of stress twice?

The basic plan of the USMLE exams is concept-based questions. There are very few if any factual ones—more on Step 1 and practically none on Step 2.

Unlike for the Indian exams, concentrating on text-based factual data is suicide. Reading the text material is just to give that "bird's eye view" of what you should have already mastered during MBBS and to familiarize yourself with subject material that has been forgotten over the years.

So doing these multiple choice based questions is apt for the USMLE prep. It keeps the mind ticking and in the exam mode constantly.

4. TIMETABLE FOR PREPARATION

Draw up a timetable and try sticking to it as much as you can. Roughly, let's say you have a three to four months schedule, and assuming you are free to study for the whole day, try out this pattern. It is important to note that the time periods mentioned below are highly variable depending on your knowledge base.

Approximately,
- Anatomy - one week
- Physiology - two weeks
- Biochemistry - one week
- Microbiology - one week
- Pharmacology - two weeks
- Behavioral sciences - one week
- Pathology - two weeks

This takes up 60 to 70 days and in the remaining month do a revision with the following idea:
- Anatomy 2-3 days
- Physiology 6 days
- Biochemistry 4-5 days
- Microbiology 4 days
- Pharmacology 6 days
- Behave sciences 2 days
- Pathology 6-8 days

Two important points to note are using Kaplan Q bank subjectwise questions after finishing each subject, and optionally, using the Kaplan Video lectures.

In accordance with what has been extensively spoken about, try and accommodate as many MCQs as possible, side by side, within this period and sprinkle MCQ days in between throughout, so that when you take the exam, in about three and a half to four months, you should have done around 20 days worth of MCQs cumulatively.

5. SUBJECTWISE PREPARATION

Anatomy

One of the very low yield topics on the test. Spend as little time as you can on it. Don't start with Anatomy. It may then be tempting to give it a thorough reading which is totally unnecessary.

The Kaplan notes are pretty much adequate. The high yield topics in Anatomy are Neuro-anatomy *and* Embryology to a certain extent.

It's correlation Anatomy that's important—for instance, you have to know anatomy of the brachial plexus or the nerve supply of the lower limb so as to understand the manifestations of different kinds of nerve palsies.

Some of the image-based questions that appear on the test are anatomy based. Utilize Webpath's resources and get a good look at the dissected specimens on the site; especially the Neuro-anatomy images and the orientation of abdominal organs. The experience certainly helps. Also, have a go at the radiology pictures. Be familiar with all the common diagnostic images.

Other than the Q series MCQs there is no need to do anymore.

Physiology

Physiology is fairly well tested, especially in correlation with Pathology.

Kaplan notes are good for Physiology and the core concepts are put forward in a lucid and easy to understand format. Give the notes a thorough reading which will be adequate for the text part.

The physiology pretest is a good source of MCQs especially when considered along with its exhaustive explanations. Try out the MCQs on BRS at the end of each chapter and the Ganong MCQs at the end of the book. These are again, the extras. The Q series should be good enough for people working under a time crunch.

Behavioral Sciences

This is the topic which has proved time and again to be the nemesis of Indian USMLE takers.

As already mentioned, whatever your test may or may not have, BS is omnipresent.

There are a few hurdles which make tackling these questions a Herculean task.
1. The Indian syllabus hardly deals with any such aspect of medical education and our exposure to the same is almost nil.
2. In the US, behavioral sciences and ethical dilemmas are well and truly a significant part of a doctor's daily life.
3. There are very few books on the topic which give you the feel of having acquired an adequate knowledge base to tackle the exam.
4. The vague and equivocal nature of the questions and the answer choices further complicates the problem. Logic does play a role, but again at least three of the answers will seem equally logical!

So what does one do?

As ever try and make the best use of the resources available. Going through whatever material there is on BS is a must. Kaplan notes are just about okay for BS. The Kaplan audio lecture on BS is particularly helpful. Read the BRS book and work out the MCQs at the end of each chapter.

Along with the Q series MCQs try as much as possible to do the pretest on BS.

The idea is to build a thought process which can filter out the frills and pick up key clues.

You will be more confident that you can get it right, and the ability to pick out the wrong answers will increase manifold.

Biochemistry

The Kaplan lectures and notes are irreplaceable.

Add to that a healthy dose of Kaplan Q bank Biochem which comes along with the much needed genetics and it's possible to virtually fall in love with the subject if done the right way. But beware, if there is a time crunch, Biochem can be quite a nightmare. Get it out of the way as soon as you can.

The subject as such is low to mid yield on the exams, so don't sweat too much if you are not interested. With Kaplan notes in hand it's quite a pleasure when you realize the rapid pace at which the author clears the air of pseudo murkiness surrounding Biochem.

There is hardly any need to go through the famed Lippincott's manual, though it is quite a good book. Try it out if you are familiar with and have used it as the reading material in the first year.

Genetics/Molecular biology is a different cup of tea altogether. Again, the problems faced are the same as that of the ones in BS.

We have little, if any, exposure and there is no particular book which gives the basic concepts in a form that's concise enough for the MLE. The pretest genetics is not adequate. That said, the situation is not as bad as it may seem, because the constancy with which BS appears on the exam is never the same for Molecular biology. Often, there are only stray questions and the unlucky may get a bunch. All I can say is—keep the fingers crossed and hope you can make up in the other sections.

Do not waste any time trying to read up a lot of molecular biology and certainly don't waste time breaking your head over those questions in the exam. Take your best shot and move on quickly.

Microbiology

Another medium yield material for the test, but tests your memory like no other.

Kaplan notes are good for priming and to an extent you can risk it to the exams with just that, along with their Q series.

For the enthusiastic, Pretest has a pretty good collection. Do try and complete the MCQs on the Jawetz review.

Though it may be difficult for most people to use the Jawetz text as reading material, the immunology part is rather good. Kaplan immunology, many felt as inadequate but personally I'm tempted to disagree. If you are planning on reading the whole of Jawetz, make sure you stick to it.

38 Acing the USMLE and the Match

Lippincott has brought out a book on Microbiology in the same Biochem/Pharm style which looks good. There is also the one in the market called "Microbiology made ridiculously simple". This one is fun to read and has comical pictures and useful mnemonics.

Always remember, stick to one book and give the others a quick review if you have the time.

Pharmacology

Next to Patho-Physiology and BS, this is the most high yield topic and some exams have appeared with a predominant Pharm base.

Always go prepared for that eventuality

For someone who has the time and money to get and use Lippincott, it wouldn't be a bad idea to supplement Kaplan notes with Lippincott, albeit using Kaplan as the primary study source.

For the strong hearted people who have the time, the recommendation is to go for the Katzung review. If you can read through and recollect at least 75% of Katzung, you can certainly rest in peace. It has enormous potential in helping with the Step 2 and the Indian exams too. In case you feel it will erode through your much valued time, try and do at least the multiple choice review questions at the end of the book.

Pathology

One of the few subjects where one can possibly skip Kaplan notes.

Go for Goljan's review of Pathology instead. Might take a while to read but it's worth the effort. It deals not just with Pathology but with integrated Patho-Physiology, which is without doubt the most tested topic on the exam. If you find it tough to handle, make some alterations on the time schedule and cut down on less tested topics like Anatomy, Biochemistry and Microbiology. The book will be of good help while taking the Indian exams too.

Goljan's lecture series is highly impressive and recommended. The man is a fantastic teacher. Get hold of the lecture audio CDs and complement those with the notes. This package should be adequate for Pathology.

For the MCQs there is massive amount of material and though most of it is worth a ton it may not be practically possible to work out the whole lot.

Along with the Kaplan Q series, try out Goljan's CD material which has 300 extremely valuable questions.

Acing the USMLE Step 1

The Pathology Pretest and the questions on the Webpath CD/website are virtual treasure troves. Then there is also the Robbins MCQ supplement which with its great pictures and conceptual questions makes a pleasurable read.

The BRS series gets submerged under this avalanche of material and can well be skipped, so can the high yield series if you have done Goljan.

There will be a few questions based on Pathology images. Scan through the pictures in Robbins once or twice, concentrating on the commoner disease entities.

Summarizing, do the Goljan book and audio lectures, Goljan and Kaplan MCQs.

Time permitting, don't miss out on the web path MCQ, which offers a pretty vast question base. Don't get bogged down or awed by the volume, just relax with and enjoy the stuff on these whenever you can.

It is not mandatory to complete the whole of Webpath since the objective is to familiarize oneself with the visual content and the histo-pathology type questions in Pathology.

6. DON'T MISS THESE!

As mentioned earlier, the other subjects that are commonly tested but missed are Immunology, Genetics, Cell Biology, Molecular Biology, Acid-base balance, Nutrition, Bio-statistics and HIV-AIDS. The High-yield series of books for these subjects are more than sufficient when it comes to these often missed subjects. They may make the difference between a 95th and a 99th percentile on the USMLE Step 1.

7. QUESTION BANKS AND CONSOLIDATED SOURCES

The Pretest clinical vignettes for Step 1 compiles questions from the other Pretest series books and can be given a go if the latter has not been attempted. It will assuredly be of good value for the exam.

The First Aid series is a well known rapid review book. If you have gone through the material mentioned above, there is no necessity to use this. It is primarily meant as a rapid revision tool for the US students who take the exam in quite a hurry. If there is a day or two to spare before the exam have a look at it. It's a proven book and might help.

BSS is yet another, but with a difference. It's integrated MCQs on the basic sciences are system based and very good. The tough part is that it runs into three volumes. Keep doing BSS once in a while in between preparation as part of the MCQs deal and don't worry too much about finishing the whole stuff.

Whatever you gain is a bonus.

Also available is the Kaplan simulated test which most students take just before the exam. I would advise you to do it too, albeit with a word of caution. It's always dangerous getting your morale down at the last minute and sometimes the simulated, being a bit on the tougher side does just that. People even vouch for the NMS series of MCQs, but frankly one just cannot afford to do everything!

Lastly, the prep discussion on Step 1 will not be complete if I don't mention the online Kaplan Q bank material which is in the form of MCQs, 2000 of them at that.

Watch out for the USMLE World USMLE Step 1 Q bank which is currently being developed. It's been receiving rave reviews from test takers, especially from the West. An elaborate discussion will follow in the Step 2 segment.

To conclude, it is very important to take the exam at the right time. All too often, applicants take the exam without adequate preparation with a false sense of confidence only to realize to their disdain, when their score is reported. Even more common is procrastination. Delaying the exam date and eligibility period until one acquires "complete mastery of all the subjects" and "super confidence" are just myths that such people never realize. We have discussed the time-tested strategies for you to assess whether you are ready to take the exam or not. So take the exam, come what may, sooner or later!

Acing the USMLE Step 2CK (Clinical Knowledge)

Paari Murugan

1. INTRODUCTION

Step 2 assesses whether you can apply medical knowledge, skills, and understanding of clinical sciences essential for the provision of patient care under supervision and includes emphasis on health promotion and disease prevention. Step 2 ensures that due attention is devoted to principles of clinical sciences and basic patient-centered skills that provide the foundation for the safe and competent practice of medicine.

Preparing for Step 2 needs more perseverance and diligence. There are conflicting opinions but there is no clear answer about which is the tougher of the two. In the same breath, also more interesting since whatever little factual element there is in Step 1 is done with and totally replaced by analytical, logical, correlative and conceptual data. There are hardly any direct questions. The time period that is required for preparation is a bit more than what you have put in for Step 1.

2. WHAT ARE THE SUBJECTS TESTED?

These are the core subjects tested for Step 2, the detailed syllabus of which is given on the USMLE web site.
- Medicine
- Surgery
- OG
- Pediatrics

- Psychiatry
- Ethics/biostatistics

3. WHAT STUDY MATERIALS TO USE?

As for any USMLE exam, stick to one set of core study materials and do a lot of MCQs. The Step 2 CK exam is no exception. The Kaplan lecture notes for each subject along with the Kaplan Q bank and Q book with First Aid as a final consolidated revision has worked for many applicants and is a time-tested study strategy. As for the other steps, your score on the Kaplan simulated exam, NBME self-assessment test and the USMLE Sample materials will give you a fair idea as to whether you are ready to take the exam or not.

4. TIME-TABLE FOR PREPARATION

A tentative schedule

- Medicine eight weeks
- Surgery one week
- OG one week
- Pediatrics one week
- Psychiatry one week
- Eth/ biostats 2-3 days

As for revision

- Medicine 10 days
- Surgery 5 days
- OG 5 days
- Pediatrics 5 days
- Psychiatry 3 days
- Ethics 2 days

The whole thing comes to around four months and you can put in at least 20 days for MCQs which should be done like suggested for Step 1, side by side.

5. SUBJECTWISE PREPARATION

Medicine

The emperor of all we had beheld for the past half a dozen years, without a shade of doubt. USMLE 2 duly acknowledges the fact. This is obviously the most tested segment on the exam and it's the ultimate test of the cumulative knowledge you have gained in the clinical years.

CMDT is the most comprehensive textbook on medicine. The book is a must as ready referral while studying for the exam but it's way beyond the scope of a regular student to go through the whole of it in the context of USMLE prep. Nevertheless, make sure all the common and off-tested topics are read and reread from this amazing book which has so much to offer.

Use Kaplan notes as core material because Medicine is too vast and one is often in the dark on where to start. Keep juggling it with CMDT and try making notes on the Kaplan book for later revision.

Do the medicine MCQs from day 1 as unlike in Step 1 you do not need a refresher course.

There are a multitude of MCQs books on Medicine but not that many based on the USMLE style. You can do the Kaplan Q series and the NMS series.

Though it is quite advanced for the Step 2 level, working on the Harrison Pretest and reading the explanations will boost your confidence up no end and give a lot of vital background info. The book is meant to be used by exam going Medicine postgraduates, so don't bother much if your head starts swimming a wee bit!

An extra plus is that the Harrison Pretest helps a lot if you plan to take up the Indian exams. Another useful study source is the Kaplan Video lectures for Medicine which are well made and can be a good mode of revision.

Surgery

As far as surgery is concerned, in plain speak—just forget everything you have learnt as an Indian medical graduate. The USMLE tests you only on management based emergency surgical care, burns, post-op, fluid management, accident/trauma care and the likes.

They are least bothered about the theoretical or for that matter practical soundness in operative procedures.

The Kaplan notes focuses exactly on the tested aspects. There are very few questions on specialty subjects like ENT and Ophthal, again on emergencies, like for example: occlusion of the ophthalmic artery and management.

For the MCQs it's the usual routine, no extra books—do Q bank and Q book and the Pretest if possible.

OG

OG is a high yield topic for Step 2 and Kaplan notes quite adequately deals with almost everything that may be tested on the exams. Give it a thorough reading and use COGDT for references.

Do the Q series, and use Pretest for that extra edge.

Pediatrics

Some of the exam days do contain a lot of the Pediatric stuff. So give it due importance. There are few books other than Kaplan that are worth-mentioning.

For the MCQs, it's the Q series and pretest. The Pediatrics Pretest is quite valuable.

Try getting hold of more MCQ resources for Pediatrics. The NMS review book and its MCQ series may be helpful.

Psychiatry

Like its Step 1 counterpart BS, Psychiatry is again the villain of the piece in Step 2. Kaplan notes are not adequate since you will get a number of ambiguous questions.

The suggestion is to read the BRS Psychiatry book which will do a lot of good.

The Psychiatry pretest is a great source to spend time with and do take care not to miss it.

Ethics/Biostats

Akin to the previous subject this one is difficult too but whatever ethics Kaplan deals with is enough for two reasons—
1. There is hardly any other book which talks on American medical ethics
2. At some point you always know it's a guess. Kaplan just gives you the feeling of having made an educated guess!

For Biostats the book available in the market is the high yield biostats, but there's nothing high yield about it. It's in a way too exhaustive for this exam's requirement.

Stick to Kaplan and get a few MCQs done from their Q series. That should do.

Keep your fingers crossed that you don't get an absolutely whacko test with millions of biostats in it!

6. DON'T MISS THESE!

Radiology, Orthopedic surgery, Trauma, Emergency Medicine, Ophthalmology, Otorhinolaryngology, Preventive Medicine and Dermatology are some topics that are commonly tested on USMLE Step two but often missed by applicants. Preparing for these off-beat topics gets you prepared to face subjects from any specialty on the exam. The short discussion of these subjects on Current Medical

Diagnosis and Treatment (CMDT) is more than sufficient to be prepared for the exam.

7. QUESTION BANKS AND CONSOLIDATED SOURCES

Like in Step 1 you have the Pretest Step 2 clinical vignettes which are nothing but a compilation from the other books.

High yield notes, Underground Clinical Vignettes and especially the Blue print series are a very good mode of revision especially when you have the time.

The online USMLE world is literally a boon to Step 2 takers and probably of more value than it is for Step 1. If one has the resources, there is no question, it is a must.

The plusses are:
1. The questions are worth their weight in gold.
2. You can take it in whatever format you want—timed, untimed or as customized test blocks on a particular subject area.
3. You can compare your performance on every question with test takers across the world in the comfort of your drawing room.
4. It helps in getting accustomed to computer-based testing.

And the minuses
1. It may not be cost effective
2. The need to be online all the time when you do the test. There is no way the material can be copied or downloaded though if you can for go real testing conditions you can work on a set test off-line and then get back online to click up the answers and read the explanations (which once loaded can be done off-line too!)

Step 2 CK USMLE world Membership:
- $90 for 30 days
- $125 for 60 days
- $175 for 90 days

The NMS question bank and the Appleton and Lange review (ALERT) are outdated and it can be said that these sources of questions are best avoided.

There is the Kaplan exam simulator like the one which was available for Step 1. A great tool for pre-exam testing. The warning on the Step 1 discussion holds good here too!

The First Aid for Step 2 can be given a wide berth, if in case there is a time constant.

Postscript

Joining a postgraduate specialty in a hurry virtually robs you of the thrill, dooming you into a one way, point of no return situation where all efforts are concentrated on to a specific aspect of medicine with the rest gradually disappearing from focus.

Moreover, it's such a joy reading from these notes as each passing day unravels the tangled mess of medical garbage that we've accumulated with such effort, replacing it with the concepts that pay due respect to our enchanting profession.

On a personal note I firmly believe in and also would like to share the message—

Enjoy the USMLE preparation. It's a cherishable experience.

The USMLE Step 2CS: How to Prepare

Dhinager Nandagopal

1. INTRODUCTION

USMLE Step 2 CS is the third exam in the series of four USMLE exams required to do residency in the US. It does create a certain amount of anxiety among IMG's as it involves interaction with patients (actually standardized patients). But preparing for Step 2CS is lot easier when compared to other USMLE exams. Ideal time to take CS is June–July. So that you will be certified at the time of application in September. Moreover you can apply for Step 3 only after you pass CS and get your ECFMG certificate. The USMLE Step 2 CS has a one year scheduling period, unlike the other Steps, and it would make sense to apply and schedule the exam early since getting test dates at your preferred test center is difficult especially in the peak season. The exam date for USMLE Step 2 CS can be rescheduled for free if done thirty days prior to the exam date, but the fee is $ 400 if rescheduled within the thirty day period. Please note that if you are applying for a B1/B2 visa for taking your Step 2 CS, you will need the Step 2 CS scheduling permit. The only positive point about the visa being rejected, if there is any, is that the Step 2 CS fee is refundable.

2. WHAT ARE THE SUBJECTS TESTED?

There are three broad areas of skills that are tested on the USMLE Step two clinical skills examination.
- Data gathering (taking a relevant History and performing a focused physical examination) (DG).
- Spoken English Proficiency (SEP).
- Communication and Interpersonal skills (IPS).

Therefore, DG+ SEP+ IPS = USMLE Step 2 CS. Step 2CS is the only exam that tests your English fluency and communication skills (before interviews). Passing Step 2 CS in the first attempt helps you to get more number of residency interviews.

3. WHAT STUDY MATERIALS TO USE?

Preparing for Step 2 CS:

As mentioned earlier, Step 2 CS is easier to prepare than other USMLE exams. Three weeks should be sufficient for the preparation. Many good sources are available in market. Top three sources include:

a. First aid for Step 2 CS
b. Kaplan Step 2 CS book.
c. Usmle World Course for USMLE Step 2 CS
d. Other courses for Step 2 CS

Let's look at each one of them and formulate a study plan.

a. First Aid for Step 2 CS

First Aid is good for Patient Note (more about it below). You can practise writing PN from FA.

b. Kaplan Step 2 CS book

Kaplan Step 2 CS book is good for improving communication and interpersonal skills.

c. Usmle World Course for USMLE STEP 2 CS

Membership for STEP 2 CS course:
- $ 50 for 30 days
- $ 60 for 45 days
- $ 70 for 60 days

USMLEWORLD is a must for CS. It also includes physical examination videos and covers all the topics required for CS. Please visit www.usmleworld.com for more information.

I would recommend you study UW thoroughly and go through FA and Kaplan if you have time. This should be enough to pass the exam. Those who don't feel confident to face the exam can attend Dr. Schwartz or Kaplan 5 day CS workshop. These are pretty expensive and can only be attended at select cities in the US.

Pros

You need not travel anywhere. It's an online preparatory course.
- Complete and comprehensive.
- Has video demonstration for history and physical.
- Best value for money.
- Most Step 2 takers are of the opinion that most cases if not all cases in their exam were from their practice case list.

Cons

Not hands-on:
- Need to find a study partner
- Need to prepare a study schedule and stick to it
- Self-preparation, so might take 2 weeks full time preparation.
  Website: www.usmleworld.com

The important thing in preparing for CS is to Practise. UW advices us to practise their course for 3 times. If you don't have a partner, you can practise in front of the mirror. The more you practise, the more you feel confident.

d. Other courses for Step 2 CS

1. *Dr Schwartz classes:* Popular course, held in New York.
   Contact info:
   Anna Lank
   212 410 8499

Day One *only*:	$ 325. US
Day Two *only*:	$ 325. US
Day One and Day Two:	$ 625. US
Day One and Day Three:	$ 725. US
Days One, Two and Three:	$ 995. US

Day 1: 8 hours History taking and communication skills
Day 2: 7-8 hours Physical exam skills
Day 3: 7-8 hours practice with standardized patients
Website: www.c3ny.org

2. Kaplan step 2 CS Live course :

Courses	Cost
Step 2 CS 6-day	$ 3299.00
Step 2 CS 5-day	$ 2799.00
Step 2 CS Practise Exam (NJMI)	$ 999.00
Step 2 CS 1-Day	
History Taking Workshop	
Physical Exam Workshop	

Pros

Comprehensive:
  Excellent tutoring
  Hands-on practise
  Best if one is in a time crunch (I know people who have taken the exam 3 days after the course and aced it).

Cons

Requires travel to the place of workshop. One needs to coordinate workshop dates with near exam dates, so advance planning is advisable.
  Website: www.kaptest.com

4. EXAM CENTER, TRAVELLING, SCHEDULING AND STANDARDISED PATIENTS

Choosing the exam center

There are only five exam centers for CS : Philadelphia, Chicago, Atlanta, Houston and LA. Philadelphia and Chicago centers get filled sooner than other centers. So, always plan well before applying for CS. It's totally false that some exam centers have higher pass rates than other. So you can choose the center which is comfortable for you.

The center locations

Clinical Skills Evaluation Center - Atlanta
Two Crown Center
1745 Phoenix Boulevard, Suite 500 (5th Floor)
Atlanta, GA 30349

Clinical Skills Evaluation Center - Chicago
8501 West Higgins Road, 6th Floor
Chicago, IL 60631

Clinical Skills Evaluation Center - Houston
400 North Sam Houston Parkway, Suite 700
Houston, TX 77060

Clinical Skills Evaluation Center - Los Angeles
100 North Sepulveda Boulevard, 13th Floor
El Segundo, CA 90245

Clinical Skills Evaluation Center - Philadelphia
3624 Market Street, 3rd Floor
Philadelphia, PA 19104

Travelling to the test center

1. By Air: For the cheapest bargain air tickets,
   - Book early.
   - Check websites like priceline, expedia, etc., compare the rates. Once you have finalized on the airline, go to the airline's website and book it directly from there. This will help you save on the fee you pay the service provider.
   - Based on your location in the US familiarize yourself with low budget flights operating in your area. For example Southwest, Continental, etc. have excellent deals to offer if flying in places in the Midwest.
   - Some cities will have 2 or more airports. And some airlines will fly to one or the other; therefore, choose carefully. For example, in Houston, Southwest flies to Hobby airport which is quite a distance from the center, therefore choose Continental airlines which flies to George Bush international airport which is closer to the exam center.
   - Always use the airport shuttle when available. It's cheaper than the cab.
   - While looking for accommodation, check with them about airport pickup and drop service. This will save you a lot. Such places will also drop you at the exam center. You will save a lot on cabs.

If you are driving

- It helps immensely if you have an international driver license. One of the first things you can do is download a copy of the driving manual for your state online and familiarize yourself with the rules. And then "simply enjoy the ride" (tip: e.g. for Indiana state driving license—simply google—easiest way to find out).

- For directions— the ultimate is a navigator like Tom-Tom, otherwise a print out from map quest or google maps from your start point to destination is an absolute must.
- Getting lost in those highways is one of the easiest things you can do in the USA.
  Other options of travel will be using the Amtrak or bus services.
  The ECFMG information booklet gives you a lot of info.
  (http://www.ecfmg.org/usmle/step2cs/centers.html)

Results

If there could be something worse than the fear of taking the exam it's waiting for the results. For the CS, the timeframe for reporting the results can vary from 3 weeks (3 Wednesdays) to sometimes 3 months. Hence it's important here for me to stress taking it as early as possible even before your other steps, so you don't get delayed with obtaining ECFMG certification.

If Step 2 CS is the last exam you are taking towards getting ECFMG certified, don't be surprised to get a FedEx first with your ECFMG certificate rather than your score report if you have passed.

If you can't still hold yourself till you get either, there is a trick commonly used called the "oasis trick". This can be used for Step 1 and 2CK as well.
1. Go to the ECFMG OASIS page. Enter your user name and password.
2. Go to score reporting to find out if your score report has been updated (it gets updated every Wednesday).
3. Next go to the interactive web application (IWA) page on ECFMG and try to apply again for the Step 2 CS. If it does not allow you to take the exam— congratulations you did it! You passed.
4. If it does allow you to take the exam, don't despair yet, wait out the days from hell, till your score report comes to be absolutely sure. Because, in the OASIS trick, if you cannot retake, you absolutely passed. If you can retake it, it isn't absolute that you didn't make it through.

Standardized patients

All the patients with whom you will be interacting in the exam are not true patients. They are actors trained by ECFMG. They score you in three categories: Integrated clinical encounter (ICE), Communication and Interpersonal Skills (CIS) and Spoken English Proficiency (SEP). It is necessary to pass all three subcomponents in order to obtain an overall passing outcome on Step 2 CS.

On the day of exam

Be at the exam center before 8 am. Take a white coat, stethoscope and the scheduling permit with you.

There will be 12 SP's on the exam. You have 25 minutes for each SP—15 minutes for clinical encounter and 10 minutes to write PN. After first 5 SP's, they provide lunch. After the next 4 SP's, they give 15 minutes break and then finish the remaining 3 cases.

In the 15 minutes of clinical encounters, you have to elicit history, do a relevant physical examination and counsel the SP. Soon after finishing the clinical encounters, you have to write/type the patient note in the computer. PN includes history, physical examination, investigation and differential diagnosis. I would recommend you write the PN because the space provided for PN in paper is less than that in computer. Don't worry about the handwriting. But it should be understandable.

Maintain your cool throughout the exam. Speak slowly. SP's also speak slowly and I did not find American accent in their speech. You will not have any problem in understanding them. If they are rude to you, don't feel bad. They are just acting under the instruction of ECFMG. React to them as you react to real patients in your clinic.

The key thing is passing CS is to Practice. Timed practise will be useful. Again the trick is to speak slowly and clearly while interacting with SP's.

5. GENERAL TIPS

PLAN A for STEP 2 CS

1. Plan early, if you are clear that you will complete the exam within the following year; it's not a bad idea to complete the application process and get the orange card ready. The scheduling time will be valid for 1 year and the fee is refundable.
2. The preparation time required for the CS can vary on how many hours you can devote each day. With full time, committed preparation it's possible to prepare in a 2 week period. The key is 3Ps - practise, practise and practise. This is assuming that the IMG has a good command over English.
3. Practise reading and analyzing.
4. practise History and physical examination.
5. practise writing the case sheet within allotted time.

6. CONSOLIDATED SOURCES AND FORUMS

Forums commonly used:
    www.usmle.net
    www.prep4usmle.com
    Web blog most useful:
    http://csprotocol.blogspot.com/

Pros

Cheaper

Cons

Will require probably 2 weeks to prepare:
- Need to find a study partner.
- No videos attached.
- Step 2 CS is a one-day exam that consists of simulated clinical encounters.
- Step 2 CS testing session lasts approximately eight hours.

REFERENCES

http://www.usmle.org/step2cs/CSECAddresses.htm

[6] The USMLE Step 2CS: High Yield Notes

Jayashree Sundararajan

1. SAMPLE CASE SHEET TO BE USED IN THE EXAM

If you can master writing this format in 7 minutes you will feel very comfortable during the actual exam. I would recommend that you print out the form from the CD that ECFMG sends you and practise on it so that you get used to the time constraint.

Head: Normocephalic, atraumatic.

Eyes: PERLA, EOM intact, no eyeball prominence.

Fundoscopic exam: No papilledema, sharp disc margin, normal vasculature.

Ear: No discharge, no edema, cerumen + intact tympanic membrane.

Nose: No congestion, no polyps, no discharge.

Throat: No tonsillar enlargement, no exudates no erythema.

Mouth: No lesions, no vesicle, no oral thrush.

Neck: No cervical lymph node enlargement, supple.

Mental Status Exam

- Patient appears well groomed.
- Alert, oriented to place person time.
- Memory intact.
- Attention and concentration intact (tested by spelling "world" backwards).
- Mood is depressed, affect consistent with mood.

- Speech fluent and goal directed.
- No hallucinations.
- No delusions.
- No suicidal/homicidal ideations.
- Insight: intact.

Neuroexam

Mental status: Alert, oriented x 3, good concentration
    CN 2 to 12: intact
    Motor: 5/5 all muscle group
    DTR: 2+ intact, symmetric
    Sensory: intact to light touch, sharp and dull
    Cerebellar: Romberg (-) finger to nose intact
    Babinski (-)
    Kernig (-) Brudenski (-)

Upper limb exam

	Lt	rt
Motor	5/5	5/5
Light touch	5/5	5/5
Sharp and dull	5/5	5/5
DTR	5/5	5/5

Lower limb

	Lt	rt
Motor	5/5	5/5
Light touch	5/5	5/5
Sharp and dull	5/5	5/5
DTR	5/5	5/5
Babinski	-	-

Respiratory system

Breathing unlaboured, Respiratory rate:
- Chest clear to auscultation, no ronchi, no wheezing
- No dullness on percussion
- No tenderness on palpation
- VF : WNL

- Chest expansion : WNL
- No cyanosis no clubbing
- Cardiac exam: S1 S2 heard,RRR, No MRG
- CVS Exam
- BP HR
- No cyanosis, no clubbing, no pedal edema
- Pulses +++ B/L
- S1 S2 (+), RRR, no MRG
- No JVD
- PMI not displaced
- Chest: clear to auscultation
- No tenderness on palpation

Abdominal exam

- Inspection: No scar, no skin changes, no redness
- Auscultation: normal BS x 4Q
- Percussion: Tympanic x 4 Q
- Palpation: No tenderness, no masses, no organomegaly
- CVA tenderness (-)
- Obturator sign (-)
- Murphys sign (-)
- Psoas sign (-)
- Rebound tenderness (-)
- Shoulder Exam (any joint exam).

	Right	*Left*
Inspection:	No redness	No redness
	No skin changes	No skin changes
Palpation:		
Tenderness	+/-	+/-
ROM	WNL	WNL
Motor strength	5/5	5/5
Sensory	5/5	5/5
Reflex	WNL	WNL
Pulses	++++	++++

Adsons test: -ve

Thyroid Exam

- Inspection: No scar, no redness
- Auscultation: No bruit
- Palpation: No tenderness, no nodules
- Hair strength: WNL
- No tremor
- Pulse: ++++ B/L
- DTR: ++++ B/L
- No pitting edema
- No thyroid exam is complete without a quick CVS assessment.
- CVS exam: S1 S2 +, RRR, No MRG

2. WHAT TO DO IN EACH STATION?

A general case history checklist:

Introducing yourself

Tips:

1. Remember to address your SP with the last name
2. Introduce yourself with your last name.
3. Smile and appear pleasant and make eye contact with your patient.
4. If you are going to interview the mother of a young patient, be sure to ask for the name of the child and use the name while addressing the patient and not as "baby".
5. Start your interview with an open, ended question.
6. Start with some pleasantries to make the patient comfortable.
7. It's acceptable to not offer your hand for a handshake in a hospital setting (reduces germ transmission) but it is impolite to decline if offered.
8. If you are unsure of the marital status of a lady address her as Mss. And not as Ms. Address males as Mr. followed by the last name.
9. After you introduce yourself, respect the personal privacy of your patient. Take the drape that is usually placed on your chair and hand it to the patient "Mr.Smith, it feels a little cold in here. This drape would make you feel little more comfortable. Is there anything I can do before we begin ?"

This way you don't forget to drape the patient and it will establish a good rapport and give you a chance to get comfortable as well. Pull up the chair and sit down comfortable. Standing all through your cases will be tiring.

" Good morning Mr. Smith, I am Dr. Rahul. I'll be your Doctor for today."
"What brings you to the hospital"?

Present history

Tips

1. In the blank sheet provided to you, write down the mneumonic that you are most comfortable with and glance at it occasionally to make sure you don't miss out something vital.
2. It is not allright not to make eye contact but it's allright if you have to occasionally make notes on your paper about the patient details.
3. Appear casual and not agitated.
4. Listen

The mnemonic I used:

SOCRATES

- S – Site
- O – Onset
- C – Character
- R – Radiation
- A – Aggravating symptoms
- T – Timing
- E – Exacerbating factors
- S – Severity

- *Site:* "Can you tell me where exactly you feel the pain? Can you place your hand or finger …."
- *Onset:* "When did it start? What were you doing when it started?"
- *Character:* "Can you describe the pain?"
- *Radiation:* "Do you feel your pain is moving elsewhere?"
- *Aggravating factors:* "Does anything you do make the pain worse?"
- *Timing:* "Has there been any change in your pain since it began?"
- "Do you feel your pain is related to certain times of the day?"
- *Exacerbating Factors:* "Does anything make the pain worse?"
- *Severity:* "On a scale of 1 to 10, 10 being the worst pain and 1 being no pain, can you grade the pain you are feeling?"

Past history

Mnemonic I used:
- PAM HUGS FOSSS
- Previous similar experience
- Allergies
- Medication use

- Hospitalizations
- Urine/Bowel habits
- GIT History
- Family history
- Ob/Gyn history
- Sleep
- Social history
- Sexual history

Opening line: "Now I am going to ask you a few questions regarding your past medical history."

Previous similar experience:
"Have you experienced something similar any other time?"
"What did you do when you last had this condition?"

Allergies: "Have you experienced any allergies to any medications, food or any other agents?"

Medications: "Are you currently using any medications?"
"Have you ever been on any prescription medications?"

Hospitalizations: "Have you ever been hospitalized for any condition previously?"

Urine/Bowel Habits

"Do you have any problems with passing urine?"
"Do you have any difficulty or changes in your bowel movements?"

GIT History

"Are you on any specific diet?"
"Have you noticed any change recently in your food habits?"
"Any changes in your appetite?"
"Any weight loss/gain?"

Sleep

"Any changes in your sleep pattern?"
"How long do you sleep?"
"Any frightening dreams?"

Social history

"I would like to briefly discuss your social life."

"Are you married or single?"

"What do you do for your living? Anything in your life you consider a stressor?"

"What are your hobbies?"

"Do you drink?" "How much?"

"Do you smoke or use tobacco in any form? How many per day? How long?"

"Do you use any recreational drugs or have at any time?" "What drugs?" "In what form have you used them?" "Have you used injectable forms?"

Note

For suspected heavy alcohol users:

CAGE questionnaire:

C – "Have you tried to cut down your alcohol consumption ever?"

A – "Have you felt annoyed when others have asked about your drinking?"

G – "Have you ever had guilt feelings about your alcohol drinking?"

E – "Do you have to have an eye opener—alcohol when you wake up?"

"Have you ever considered quitting?"

"Have you attempted quitting?"

For cigarette users

Always advise and broach on the subject of quitting and offer help. If they refuse then proceed with your interview, but remember to again touch and offer counseling at the end of your patient encounter.

Start with an open-ended question "Can you tell me more about your smoking?"

Proceed towards "When did you start? How long? Attempts to quit? Pressure to quit? Concerns about smoking affecting health? Concerns of the patient towards family, passive smoking?"

"If you are interested in quitting you are free to approach me. Help me to help you quit smoking. Think about it and I will ask the nurse to provide you with information booklets on smoking cessation. We will talk about it when you feel ready."

Sexual History

"Now, can I ask you a few questions pertaining to your sexual life. It is very important to get a complete picture of your current health status. I assure you that the information you provide will be kept strictly confidential. Can I proceed?"

"Are you sexually active?"

"Is your sexual partner male or female?"

"Do you have multiple sexual partners?"

"Do you use any form of contraception?"

"Do you use condoms?" "Do you use them regularly?"

"Do you have any problems in your sexual life you would want to discuss?"

"Have you ever been diagnosed or treated for any sexually transmitted diseases?"

"Have you been tested for HIV?"

After you have finished the major part of your interview, proceed towards physical exam. Remember you can always ask questions during the physical exam. Balance your interview with time.

"Mr. Smith, I would now like to proceed with giving you a physical exam."

"Is there anything else you would like to discuss with me that you feel pertains to your condition before we proceed".

Ask this question while you wash your hands. This way you give an opportunity for the SP to ask you a challenging question as well as add important information in the history you may have missed.

Wash your hands with warm water; this will warm your hands. Do not forget to wash your hands. I still remember the first advice from my seniors who had taken the exam "Knock the door, wash your hands and drape. You will pass."

2. LIST OF CASES COMMONLY TESTED IN THE EXAM

CNS

1. Case of dizziness
2. Case of forgetfulness
3. Case of fainting spells
4. Case of an elderly patient complaining of arm / leg weakness
5. Elderly patient C/O frequent falls
6. Pt C/O loss of hearing/vision
7. Pt C/O ringing sensation in ears
8. Elderly patient with sleeplessness
9. Elderly patient with frequent/difficulty micturition
10. Pt with seizures
11. Pt with headache.

CVS

1. Case of chest pain
2. Case of breathlessness
3. Case of palpitations.

RS

1. Case of persistent cough
2. Case of hemoptysis
3. Patient with H/O sickle cell disease with chest pain/ joint pain
4. Patient with C/O sore throat.

Abdomen

1. Case of abdominal pain
2. Case of malena
3. Case of a 27 year old with hematuria
4. Case of a 27 year old with persistent diarrhea/acute diarrhea
5. Case of constipation
6. Patient with epigastric pain/abdominal pain
7. Case of hematomesis.

Joints

1. Case of a heavy weight lifter with hip pain
2. Case of a 56 year old lady with generalized bone pain
3. Case of a patient with shoulder pain
4. Patient with low back pain.

Ob/Gyn

1. Counseling a patient with trichomonas
2. Case of amenorrhea
3. Patient with vaginal bleed
4. Patient with breast tenderness.

Pediatrics

1. Case of a 1 year old with fever
2. Case of a 1 year old with rash
3. Case of a 1 year old with vomiting
4. Case of a fussy baby

5. Bed wetting
6. Teenager with vomiting and rt lower quadrant pain.

Psychiatry

1. Panic attacks
2. Case of hallucinations/ hearing voices
3. Case of pt with addiction (alcohol /drugs/ tobacco/ cigarettes)
4. Smoking cessation counseling
5. Depression.

Skin

1. Patient C/O yellowish discoloration of skin
2. Patient C/O rash
3. Patient C/O of insect bite.

Telephone conversation

Mother with a child at home with fever without means of transportation.

Miscellaneous

1. Patient with night sweats and weight loss
2. Counseling a patient newly diagnosed with HTN/DM
3. Patient visit for pre-employment health check up
4. Case of impotence
5. A young lady with bruises
6. Patient for HIV follow up
7. Obesity counseling
8. Breaking bad news.

REFERENCES

www.usmle.net
www.usmleforum.com

Acing the USMLE Step 3

Dhinager Nandagopal

1. INTRODUCTION

Step 3 assesses whether you can apply medical knowledge and understanding of biomedical and clinical sciences essential for the unsupervised practice of medicine, with emphasis on patient management in ambulatory settings. Step 3 provides a final assessment of physicians assuming independent responsibility for delivering general medical care.

Step 3 is the fourth and final exam in the USMLE series. Programs will be happy to call you for an interview if you have cleared Step 3. Moreover you should have cleared Step 3 before match day in order to get a H-1B visa and Step 3 is required to get state medical license. The official link is listed at the end of the book and it would be useful to read it before beginning to prepare for the exam.

Step 3 is a two day exam

Day 1: 7 blocks 48 MCQs each, 1 hour for each block.
Day 2: 4 blocks of 38 MCQs each, 45 min for each block.
Followed by 9 CCS cases, maximum of 25 minutes for each case.

The MCQs in Step 3 are longer and trickier than in Step 2 CK. None of the MCQ source out there in market resembles actual exam MCQs but UW is close to the exam. Ethics and statistics are heavily tested on Step 3. Most of the questions are from Internal Medicine.

Clinical case simulations

Always keep an eye on the time as one has to rush through last few questions in most of the blocks. Questions in Step 3 are general. Most of the questions were like: a patient comes to your clinic with fever, what will you suggest? Tepid sponging or Antipyretics? Both of them are correct but you have to choose one from them. For more than 80% of the questions one is not sure of the answer. But they test only common conditions like those which you can see in your clinic.

American graduates take Step 3 usually in second year of residency. More over Step 3 is designed to be taken during residency. Without hands-on clinical experience in US, IMG's feel Step 3 to be difficult. In fact, Step 3 is the most difficult of all Usmle exams. But the good thing is you only need to pass (>75) Step 3 and CCS helps us to pass the exam.

Step 3: This exam cannot be taken unless you are ECFMG certified. The advantage of taking Step 2 CK last truly shows here. If you follow the pattern of Step 1, 2 CS then CK, you will have your results within 4 weeks and get your ECFMG certificate around that time too if all your transcripts have been verified. It would take another, maximum 3 weeks for you to apply and get the permit to take Step 3. It is possible to continue your preparation for Step 3 within that 7 week period so you don't lose any time and you will be able to take the exam in 7 weeks with time enough for an ideal preparation. It also helps because Step 3 is an extended preparation from Step 2 materials with exam format changes. Though it would not hurt to have a high score in Step 3, it's more of a formality in getting a H-1 B visa and a state license. Therefore for many it might be a race against time to get this exam over within the last leg of journey towards getting into a residency program.

2. WHAT ARE THE SUBJECTS TESTED?

The USMLE website says it all: Step 3 is an assessment of the test-taker's ability to apply basic science and clinical science medical knowledge to the unsupervised practice of Medicine. Hence all the subjects tested on the other Steps, with a particular emphasis on Internal Medicine, especially in the ambulatory setting is a feature of the exam.

3. WHAT STUDY MATERIALS TO USE?

I would recommend the following materials for preparation for USMLE Step 3:
1. Kaplan Step 2 CK notes or Kaplan Step 3 notes
2. Swanson's Family Practice Review
3. MCQs in USMLE World, Kaplan Q bank and Kaplan Q book

4. First Aid for the USMLE Step 3
5. Computerized Case Simulations (CCS)—FSMB CD, USMLE World CCS Cases
6. FSMB CD MCQs and Kaplan simulated exam (to assess readiness for real exam)

The cost of the courses for Step 3 available on USMLE World:

Step 3 MCQs Only Membership

- $95 for 30 days
- $105 for 45 days
- $125 for 60 days
- $175 for 90 days

Step 3 CCS Only Membership

- $40 for 30 days
- $50 for 45 days
- $60 for 60 days
- $70 for 90 days

Step 3 MCQs + CCS Membership

- $125 for 30 days
- $140 for 45 days
- $160 for 60 days
- $185 for 90 days

4. TIME TABLE FOR PREPARATION

Two months of preparation should be enough to clear Step 3, as scores are not important. But if you had taken Step 2 CK long back, then you would require more time to prepare for Step 3.

The most commonly used materials are the Kaplan Step 2 CK notes followed by First Aid for Step 3. Even though USMLE Step 3 notes are available; most people feel that it is not as comprehensive as the Step 2 CK notes. Swanson's Family Practise Review is more a source of information than a source of questions but is highly recommended considering that the bulk of Step 3 MCQs are based on Family Practise. The sources of questions are the Kaplan Q bank and Q book. The unique aspect of the Step 3 exam is the CCS, for which practice is the most important tool in preparation. The USMLEWORLD CCS and the FSMB CD are more than enough for the CCS. It is important to be comfortable using the software for the CCS using the FSMB CD.

The easiest and time-tested method to familiarize oneself with the software is to try to "kill" the patient as soon as possible by typing in all the wrong orders and then work backwards to make the patient better. A common mistake made by IMGs is concentrating too much on the CCS and not on the MCQs even though MCQs compose 3/4 of the exam. Also note that the failure rate in USMLE Step 3 is very high among IMGs especially those without US clinical experience. A few months of USCE can make a lot of difference when you take Step 3 since the exam is set entirely in the US practice setting. Since Step 3 tests your basic and clinical science knowledge applied in the unsupervised practice of Medicine, it is too vast to be mastered in a few months of preparation; it is more about how much you already know rather than how much you can learn.

One week before the exam test yourself with USMLE Step 3 sample questions and NBME questions (go to NMBE.org); go through University of Washington ethic's website once before you go for exam.

REFERENCES

http://www.usmleworld.com/step3pricing.asp

The USMLE Step 3: High Yield Notes

Muralikrishna G

The USMLE Step 3 exam is composed of two major parts: MCQs and the CCS. As far as the MCQs are concerned, the reader is advised to use the study materials suggested in the chapter on how to prepare for the USMLE Step 2. This section will focus exclusively on the widely popular one hundred golden rules for dealing with the section on CCS.

100 GOLDEN RULES FOR CCS CASES

1. If a patient has a fever, give acetaminophen (unless it is contraindicated).
2. If a patient is on a statin or you order a statin, get baseline LFTs and check frequently.
3. If a patient is found to have abnormal LFTs, get a TSH levels.
4. If a patient is going to surgery (including cardiac catheterization), make them NPO.
5. All NPO patients must also have their urine output measured (type "urine output").
6. If a woman is between 12 and 52 years of age and there is no mention of a very recent menses (that is, < 2 weeks ago), order a beta-hCG.
7. Don't forget to discontinue anything that is no longer required (especially if you are sending the patient home).
8. When a patient is stable, decide whether or not you should change locations (if you anticipate that the patient could crash in the very near future, send the patient to the ICU; if the patient just needs overnight monitoring, send to the ward; if the patient is back to baseline, send home with follow-up).

9. In any diabetic (new or long-standing), order an HbA1c as well as continuous accuchecks.
10. If this is a long-standing diabetic, also order an ophthalmology consult (to evaluate for diabetic retinopathy).
11. In any patient with respiratory distress (especially with low oxygen saturations), order an ABG.
12. In any overdose, do a gastric lavage and activated charcoal (no harm in doing so, unless the patient is unconscious or has risk for aspiration).
13. In any suicidal patient, admit to ward and get "suicide contract" and "suicide precautions".
14. Patients who cannot tolerate aspirin get Clopidogrel or Ticlopidine.
15. Post-PTCA patients get Abciximab.
16. In any bleeding patient, order PT, PTT, and Blood Type and Crossmatch (just in case they have to go to the OR).
17. In any pregnant patient, get "Blood Type and Rh" as well as "Atypical Antibody Screen".
18. In any patient with excess bleeding (especially GI bleeding), type "no aspirin" upon D/C of patient.
19. If the patient is having any upper GI distress or is at risk for aspiration, order "head elevation" and "aspiration precautions".
20. In any asthmatic, order bedside FEV 1 and PEFR (and use this to follow treatment progress).
21. Before you D/C a patient, change all IV meds to PO and all nebulizers to MDI.
22. In any patient who has GI distress, make them NPO.
23. All diabetic in-patients get accuchecks, D/C oral hypoglycemic agents, start insulin, HbA 1c, advise strict glycemic control, recommend diabetic foot care.
24. All patients with altered mental status of unknown etiology get a "fingerstick glucose" check (for hypoglycemia), IV thiamine, IV dextrose, IV naloxone, urine toxicology, blood alcohol level, NPO.
25. If hemolysis is in the differential, order a reticulocyte count.
26. If you administer heparin, check platelets on Day 3 and Day 5 (for heparin-induced thrombocytopenia), as well as frequent H and H.
27. If you administer coumadin, check daily PT/INR until it is within therapeutic range for two consecutive days.
28. Before giving a woman coumadin, isotretinoin, doxycycline, OCPs or other teratogens, get a beta-hCG.
29. If you give furosemide (Lasix), also give KCl (it depletes K^+).

30. All children who are given gentamycin, should have a hearing test (audiometry) and check BUN/Cr before and after treatment.
31. Don't forget about patient comfort! Treat pain with IV morphine, nausea with phenergan, constipation with PO docusate, diarrhea with PO loperamide, insomnia with PO temazepam.
32. ALL ICU patients get stress ulcer prophylaxis with IV omeprazole or ranitidine.
33. If you put a patient on complete bedrest (such as those who are pre-op), get "pneumatic compression stockings".
34. If fluid status is vital to a patient's prognosis (such as those with dehydration, hypovolemia, or fluid overload), place a Foley catheter and order "urine output".
35. If a CXR shows an effusion, get a decubitus CXR next.
36. If you intubate a patient you ALSO have to order "mechanical ventilation" (otherwise the patient will just sit there with a tube in his mouth!).
37. With any major procedure (including surgery, biopsy, centesis), you MUST type "consent for procedure" (typing consent will not reveal any results).
38. With any fluid aspiration (such as paracentesis or pericardiocentesis), get fluid analysis separately (it is not automatic). If you don't order anything on the fluid, it will just be discarded.
39. With high-dose steroids (such as in temporal arteritis), give IV ranitidine, calcium, vitamin D, alendronate, and get a baseline DEXA scan.
40. In all suspected DKA or HHNC, check osmolality and ketone levels in the serum.
41. In ALCOHOLIC ketoacidosis, just give dextrose (no need for insulin), in addition to IV normal saline and thiamine.
42. All patients over 50 with no history of FOBT or colonoscopy should get a rectal exam, a FOBT, and have a sigmoidoscopy or colonoscopy scheduled.
43. All women > 40 years old should get a yearly clinical breast exam and mammogram (if risk factors are present, start at 35).
44. All men > 50 years old should get a prostate exam and a PSA (if risk factors are present, start at 45).
45. If a patient has a terminal disease, advise "advanced directives".
46. In any patient with a chronic disease that can cause future altered mental status, type "medical alert bracelet" upon D/C.
47. Any patient with diarrhea should have their stool checked for "ova and parasites", "white cells", "culture", and C. diff antigen (if warranted).
48. Any patient on lithium or theophylline should have their levels checked.
49. All patients with suspected MI should be given a station (and check baseline LFTs).

50. All suspected hemolysis patients should get a direct Coombs test.
51. Schedule all women older than 18 for a Pap smear (unless she has had a normal Pap within one year).
52. Pre-op patients should have the following done: "NPO", "IV access", "IV normal saline", "blood type and crossmatch", "analgesia", "PT", "PTT", "pneumatic compression stockings", "Foley", "urine output", "CBC", and any appropriate antibiotics.
53. If a patient requires epinephrine (such as in anaphylaxis), and he/she is on a beta-blocker, give glucagon first.
54. If lipid profile is abnormal, order a TSH.
55. All dementia and alcoholic patients should be advised "no driving".
56. To diagnose Alzheimer's, first rule out other causes. Order a CT head, vitamin B_{12} levels, folate levels, TSH, and routine labs like CBC, BMP, LFT, UA. Also, if the history suggests it, order a VDRL and HIV ELISA as well.
57. Also rule out depression in suspected dementia patients.
58. For all women who are sexually active and of reproductive age, give folate. In fact, you should give ALL your patients a multivitamin upon D/C home.
59. All pancreatitis patients should be made NPO and have NG suction so that no food can stimulate the pancreas.
60. Send patients home on a disease-specific diet: diabetics get a "diabetic diet", hypertensives get a "low salt diet", irritable bowel patients get a "high fiber diet", hepatic failure patients get "low protein diet", etc.
61. Do not give a thrombolytic (tPA or streptokinase) in a patient with unstable angina patient.
62. Patients who are having a large amount of secretions, order "pulmonary toilet" to reduce the risk of aspiration.
63. Every patient should be advised to wear a "seatbelt", to "exercise", and advised about "compliance".
64. In any patient who presents with an unprotected airway (as in overdoses, comatoses), get a CXR to rule out aspiration.
65. In any patient with one sexually transmitted disease (such as Trichomonas), check for other STDs as well (Gonorrhea, Chlamydia, HIV, syphilis, etc.) and do a Pap smear in all women with an STD.
66. Remember to treat children with croup with a "mist tent" and racemic epinephrine.
67. Any acute abdomen patient with a suspected or proven perforation, give a TRIPLE antibiotic: Gentamycin, Ampicillin, Metronidazole.
68. Get iron studies in patients with microcytic anemia if the cause is unknown. Order "iron", "ferritin", "TIBC".

69. Women with vaginal discharge should get a KOH prep, saline (wet) prep, vaginal pH, cervical gonococcal, chlamydia culture.
70. If a woman is found to have vaginal candida, check her fasting glucose.
71. When the 5 minute warning screen is displayed, go through the following mnemonic (RATED SEX). I know it probably is not the best mnemonic, but it is difficult to forget!: Recreational drugs/Reassurance, Alcohol, Tobacco, Exercise Diet, e.g. high protein, no lactose, low fat, etc.) Seat belt/Safety plan/Suicide precautions Education ("patient education"),X (stands for safe sex).
72. All suspected child abuse patients should be admitted and you should order THREE consults: consult "child protection services", consult "ophthalmology" (to look for retinal hemorrhages), consult "psychiatrist" (to examine the family dynamics).
73. When a woman reaches menopause, she should have a "fasting lipid profile" checked (because without estrogen, the LDL will rise and the HDL will drop), a DEXA scan (for baseline bone density), and of course, FOBT and colonoscopy (if she is over 50).
74. If colon cancer is suspected, order a CEA; if pancreatic cancer, order CA 19-9; if ovarian cancer, order CA 125.
75. Remember to give "phototherapy" to a newborn with pathologic unconjugated bilirubinemia (it is not helpful if it is predominantly conjugated). Also, with phototherapy, keep the neonate on IV fluids (the heat can dehydrate them), and give erythromycin ointment in their eyes.
76. Before giving a child prednisone, get a PPD.
77. If a patient is found to have high triglycerides, check "amylase" and "lipase" (high triglycerides can cause pancreatitis).
78. Remember that any newborn under 3 weeks of age who develops a fever is SEPSIS until proven otherwise. Admit to the ward and culture Everything: "blood culture", "urine culture", "sputum culture", and even "CSF culture". And give antibiotics to cover Everything.
79. If you get a high lead level in a child, you have to check a "venous blood lead level" to confirm. If the value is > 70, admit immediately and begin IV "dimercaprol" and "EDTA". Order "lead abatement agency" and "lead paint assay" upon discharge.
80. If you perform arthrocentesis, send the synovial fluid for "gram stain" and the 3 CS: "crystals", "culture", and "cell count".
81. If a patient has exophthalmos with hyperthyroidism, it is not enough to just treat the hyperthyroidism (as the eye findings may worsen). You should give prednisone.

74 Acing the USMLE and the Match

82. If any patient has cancer, get an "oncology consult".
83. In a patient with rapid atrial fibrillation, decrease the heart rate first (then worry about converting to sinus rhythm). Use a CCB (diltiazem) or a beta-blocker (metoprolol) for rate control.
84. In any patient with new-onset atrial fibrillation, make sure you check a TSH.
85. In any patient with suspected fluid volume depletion, order "postural vitals" to detect orthostasis.
86. Before a colonoscopy or a sigmoidoscopy, you should prepare the bowel: make the patient NPO, give IV fluids (if necessary) and order "polyethylene glycol".
87. Any patient with Mobitz II or complete heart block gets an immediate "transcutaneous pacemaker". Then order a cardiology consult to implant a "transvenous pacemaker".
88. If calcium level is abnormal, order a "serum magnesium", "serum phosphorus", and "PTH".
89. Treat both malignant hyperthermia and neuroleptic malignant syndrome with "dantrolene".
90. All splenectomy patients get a "pneumovax", an "influenza" vaccine, and a "hemophilus" vaccine if not previously given.
91. If you give INH (for Tb), also give "pyridoxine" (this is vitamin B_6).
92. If you give pyrazinamide, get baseline "serum uric acid" levels.
93. If you give ethambutol, order an ophthalmology consult (to follow possible optic neuritis).
94. If you perform a thoracocentesis (lung aspirate), send the EFFUSION as well as a peripheral blood sample for: LDH and protein (to help differentiate a transudate versus an exudates) and pH of the effusion.
95. Give sickle cell disease children prophylactic penicillin continuously until they turn 5 years old.
96. Any patient with a recent anaphylactic reaction (for any reason), should get "skin test" for allergens (to help prevent future disasters) and consult an allergist.
97. Do not give cephalosporins to any patient with anaphylactic penicillin allergies (there is a 5% cross-reactivity).
98. Order Holter monitor on patients who have had symptomatic palpitations.
99. Any patient with a first-time panic attack gets a "urine toxicology" screen, a TSH, and "finger stick glucose".
100. All renal failure patients get: "nephrology consult", "calcium acetate" (to decrease the phosphorus levels), "calcium" supplement, and erythropoietin.

Section Three
Entering the United States–the Bottlenecks

Tourist Visa (B1/B2)

Dhinager Nandagopal

1. INTRODUCTION

If you thought that the USMLE exams were the toughest nuts to crack in your path to a US Residency, you are absolutely wrong. The biggest hurdle, undoubtedly and frighteningly so because it is totally not in your hands, is entering the United States. There are various routes and paths to entering the United States. We will discuss some of the commonly used routes.
1. Tourist visa (B1/B2)
2. Student visa (F1)
3. Other routes

In this section, we will discuss the option of entering the United States using the tourist visa.

2. TYPES OF A TOURIST VISA

Even though tourist visas are basically of two types, B1-the business tourist visa and B2-the actual tourist visa, here we will discuss the various ways by which a medical student or a medical graduate can get a tourist visa to enter the United States.
a. To take the USMLE Step 2 CS exam.
b. To do an Observership or an externship as a medical graduate.
c. To attend interviews at universities or hospitals in the United States for Residency.
d. To do Clinical rotations/ electives in the United States as a medical student.

Roughly speaking, as you go from a to d, the chances of getting a visa increase from 50% at *a* to nearly 100% at *d*.

An arguably foolproof method to get a B1/B2 visa is to apply at the US Consulate for attending interviews as the purpose of the trip. One can apply to universities and programs even with just one Usmle Step, and hence it is possible to get interviews from community hospitals, especially in non-competitive specialties and use it to get a B1/B2 visa.

US clinical electives: as a medical student, you can apply for a B1/B2 visa to attend a 1 or 2 month elective at a US university or hospital. The procedure to apply for an elective and get into it is discussed elsewhere in the book. Further, the US electives considerably bolster your chances of getting into competitive specialties and competitive programs.

When you first tell your relatives or friends about you desire of doing residing in the US, the first question they ask is "Will you get the visa", "It's very difficult to get visa" or something like that. Even you may be skeptical about getting a visitor's visa (B1/B2 category) to take USMLE Step 2 CS and to attend interviews in the universities. This chapter will help you relieve your anxiety about visa.

3. PROCEDURE TO BOOK AN APPOINTMENT

Before getting visa appointment

Always plan well before you get a visa appointment. Waiting time for the appointment at the US consulates in India is usually around 3-4 months. I would recommend that you go for visa interview in April–May and take USMLE Step 2 CS in June-July so that you will be ECFMG certified at the time of interviews in the universities.

To get visa appointment

For Chennai, Delhi and Kolkata regions go to www.vfs-usa.co.in. For Mumbai region go to www.visa-services.com.

4. PREPARING THE DOCUMENTS

Visa Application Forms

On the day of visa interview you need to take two visa application forms—DS 156 and DS 157. Both can be down loaded from http://travel.stage.gov/visaforms.html. While filling DS 156, its better to ask visa for 2 weeks to take USMLE Step 2 CS if you go for visa before May. If you get observership you may ask visa for 6 months but you need to show a letter from the university where you will be doing observership. If you go for visa later than July ask for visa for 6 months to take CS and to attend interviews.

Tourist Visa (B1/B2)

If you are a student, it's better to ask for visa for 2 weeks as you cannot stay in the US for 6 months while doing CRRI in India. Sponsor of the trip should be either you or your parents.

Documents

Documents which you take should complement the answers in DS 156 and 157. The following is the general list of documents which you must take with you while going for visa interview :

- Covering letter addressing. The US Consulate General. It should contain a few lines about yourself and why you are going to the US and the documents enclosed. The following are the documents:
- Visa application forms (DS 156 & 157)
- Visa appointment letter
- 1 Colour photo (5 x 5)
- Passport
- Degree Certificate
- MBBS Mark sheet
- Step 1 and 2 CK score reports.
- Visa letter from ECFMG, which you get after scheduling your Step 2 CS.
- If you are working take a letter from the hospital.
- If you are a student, take a letter from your college starting you need to come back to India to finish the course/CRRI.
- Scheduling permit for Step 2 CS.
- Auditor's (Chartered Accountant) report: It should contain both your solid and liquid assets.
- Bank statement for the past 6 months. Ideally you should have 5 + lakhs in your (or in your parents accounts if they are your sponsor) account for more than 6 months. If you need to transfer money from other accounts do it gradually. Don't do bulk transfers like 3 lakhs on a particular day.
- IT (Income Tax) returns for the past 3 years.
- I-134: It should be filled and sent to you by your relative in the US. They also should include a covering letter (stating they will take care of your expenses in the US), their employment letter and their six months bank statement.
- You can block your air ticket and take the print of your ticket and type "itinerary enclosed" in travel plan column of Dist.
- If you get Observership, take a letter from the University where you will be doing Observership.

5. PREPARING FOR THE INTERVIEW

One can be confident of getting 99's in both USMLE Steps 1 and 2 CK, but no one is confident of getting visa. To get 99 it requires a lot of time and hard work. To get visa you need to act smart in the limited amount of time. This may be less than 2 minutes. Fearing visa rejection is just a negative thought in your mind. It occurs because you visualize the misery you have to undergo if your visa gets rejected. The things you fear do not really exist except as thoughts in your mind. One famous quote goes like this: "The things I feared have come upon me". Think good and good follows. Convert forcefuly your negative thoughts into positive thoughts like "I am getting the visa, no questions about it".

Remove all skepticism about getting visa from your mind. Believe you will get the visa and you will get it. Be confident of getting the visa and prepare well for the visa interview.

- Your main task in the visa interview is to show strong ties in India and to convince the visa officer that you will come after taking the exam/interviews. Keep visiting the web site of the US Consulate for updates. Another useful time to apply for a B1/B2 visa is during your Internship when you can tell and show the visa officer that you will need to come back after taking the exam since you need to complete your internship.

On the day of Interview

Walk 25% faster to visa officer, lift your shoulders back, lift your head up. Make eye contact. SMILE. Be confident, act confidently. Answer the questions boldly and to the point. Speak slowly and clearly.

Get a balanced view of the visa officer. Remember visa officer is important but you ARE ALSO IMPORTANT. Think—we're just two important people discussing something of mutual interest & benefit.

Some common questions

- What are you doing now?
- When/where did you graduate?
- Why are you going to the US?
- How long will you stay in the US? Why 6 months?
- Who will pay for your trip?
- Will you come back?
- How will you prove you will come back?

- Why the US? Why not in India?
- What specialty will you be applying for?
- To which universities have you applied?
- Why are you taking CS?
- Why can't you take CS in India?
- What happens if you fail in CS?
- What is USMLE?
- What about Step 3?
- What will you do after finishing residency?
- How much is your annual income. If it is less than 2 lakhs they may ask how you will support yourself for 6 months in the US (for this question show 1-134).

Prepare well for the above questions and be genuine in answering all the questions. For Step 3 you may say "Step 3 is not required to join residency in the US & you will not be taking Step 3".

6. GOT MY VISA, THEN WHAT?

Once the consular officer has issued the visa, you have to pay the visa issuance fee and your passport will be couriered to you in the next seventy two hours. Celebrate! You have cleared the rate-limiting step. Depending on whether you get a single entry or a multiple entry visa, plan your trip to the US accordingly.

If you get a multiple entry visa, either a one year or a ten year visa, you can enter the United States many times; once for your USMLE Step 2 CS, once for your Observership/ externship and then for your USMLE Step 3 and interviews, as and when you please.

If you get a single entry visa, then you have to plan smart. Plan so that you will enter the United States in the beginning of July, take your Step 2 CS immediately so that you will have your Step 2 CS result and ECFMG Certificate by September 1st, then apply for and start your Observership/ Externship/ Research in the US in July-Nov. Try to take your Step 3 by October and interview at the programs that invite you in November, December and January. This plan is solid considering that you finish your USMLE Step 2 CS/ USMLE Step 3/ US Clinical experience/ Residency application and interviews in one shot. But you have to convince the visa officer at the Port of entry in the United States to issue you a six month period of stay in the United States by showing him the scheduling permit of the exam and the acceptance into an Observership or externship.

7. DID NOT GET MY VISA, THEN WHAT?

If you don't get visa
- Visa rejections can come under any one of the following categories:
- 214(b) = Potential Immigrant (not able to convince visa officer that you will come back)
- 221(g) = Insufficient documents.

Most of your rejections come under 214(b)
1. Don't lose hope. Do not waste time & energy being discouraged. Don't berate yourself.
2. Delay your next interview by 4 months. Do not allow the visa issue to hamper your preparation for Usmle Steps. Again, believe you will get visa. There is nothing wrong in believing that you will get visa in next attempt.
3. In your subsequent attempts, your answers should be similar to the one in the first attempt. They have a record of your answers in the computer and compare it with answers in subsequent attempts. So always be genuine while answering questions.
4. If you go for visa interview later than September, you can take the printouts of the (e-mail) interview call from the programs you applied for on September 1.
5. My visa got rejected six times, on my sixth attempt the visa officer was very polite and told me to come at a later date and not immediately. I was frustrated, but did not lose hope and had faith in God. Finally I got the Visa (B1/B2) in my seventh attempt.
6. Send an e-mail to ECFMG and tell them that your visa got rejected.

Student Visa (F1)

Jayashree Sundararajan

INTRODUCTION

The F1 visa is a non-immigrant student visa issued for the purpose of studying at an accredited US college or university.

Other types of student visas

J1 visa is for those who will be engaged in non-academic or vocational study or training at an institution in the US. M-1 visa is for people who will be participating in an exchange visitor program in the US. The "J" visa is for educational and cultural exchange programs.

Traditionally, post-MBBS students tend to decide to enroll in an academic course in the US, because of the lower rate of rejection of the student visa, to gain entry into the US, get an additional degree while preparing for the USMLE. Multiple course choices are available however; the commonest courses choosen are MPH (Masters in Public Health), MHA (Masters in Hospital Administration) MS (Masters in Science), Masters in Informatics, and Masters in Biomedical Engineering.

THE EXAMS: GRE, GMAT AND TOEFL

The exams required

GRE Graduate Record Examinations

The GRE General Test measures critical thinking, analytical writing, verbal reasoning, and quantitative reasoning skills that have been acquired over a long period of time and that are not related to any specific field of study.

Analytical writing

- Issue task:
- Two essay topics are presented and you choose one
- Allotted time: 45 minutes

Argument task

- No choice of topic
- Allotted time: 30 minutes

Verbal

- 30 multiple choice questions
- Allotted time: 30 minutes

Quantitative

- 28 multiple choice questions
- Allotted time: 45 minutes

GRE test fee

- 140$ US till June 30, 2006
- 160$ US from July 1, 2006

How long is the GRE score valid?

- 5 years

How to apply?

Online: To schedule a test appointment online in India, you can complete the required details online on the official GMAT registration website:

http://www.mba.com/mba/TaketheGMAT

The test fee payments for online test appointments can only be made by credit card or debit card. So, you need to have a Visa, Master Card, JCB or American Express credit card or a Visa or Master debit card to register online for the GMAT.

By Phone

To schedule your test appointment in India by phone, please call the following number:

- Telephone: **0120 4324628** (95120 from New Delhi) 9:00 a.m. to 6:00 p.m. Indian Standard Time.

By Mail or FAX

Contact the nearest USEFI center located in the US Consulate to get the GMAT information booklet and complete the registration form.

If you wish to mail your form, please send your completed form along with the appropriate payment to:

Pearson VUE
Attention: GMAT® Program
PO Box 581907
Minneapolis, MN 55458-1907
USA
Or
Fax the completed form to: +61 2 9901 3330

When to take the exam?

All-round-the-year. The test is five-days-a-week (Monday through Friday).

GMAT (Graduate Management Admission Test)

The GMAT exam consists of three main parts:
Analytical writing assessment:
The AWA consists of two separate writing tasks—Analysis of an Issue and Analysis of an Argument.
Allotted time frame: 30 minutes for each section.

The Quantitative Section

The Quantitative section consists of 37 multiple choice questions to test Data Sufficiency and Problem Solving.
Allotted time frame: 75 minutes.

The Verbal Section

The verbal section contains 41 multiple choice questions of three question types—Reading Comprehension, Critical Reasoning, and Sentence Correction.

Allotted time frame: 75 minutes
Break time: 10 minutes between each section (optional).

When to take GMAT

You can take GMAT all-round-the-year. The test is administered five-days-a-week (Monday through Friday), twice-a-day. September to December is the high season for GMAT, so in case you intend to take the test during this period, it's advisable to register at least 90 days in advance to get a date of your choice. Otherwise, registering at least 15 days in advance is mandatory. The GMAT test lasts roughly four hours, and most centers offer two slots: 9:00 a.m. and 2:00 p.m.

How long are the test scores valid?

5 years

Preparation

The Official Guide for GMAT Review—10th Edition
Published by: GMAC
Arco's Master the GMAT CAT With CD
Published by: Arco
Cracking the GMAT With CD
Published by: The Princeton Review
HOME PAGE
http://www.mba.com/mba/TaketheGMAT
WWW.GMAT.ORG
TOEFL:
Home Page: www.ets.org

Test fee

The TOEFL test fee is US $ 140 for tests taken through June 2006. The fee for testing after July 1, is US $ 150. Test of English as a Foreign Language is a standardized test that evaluates the English proficiency of people whose native language is not English.

TOEFL test is administered as a computer-based test in India. The TOEFL test is developed and administered by the US-based "Educational Testing Service" (ETS). "Prometric Testing Services Pvt. Ltd." administers the test at 9 centers in the country: **Ahmedabad, Allahabad, Bangalore, Calcutta, Chennai, Hyderabad, Mumbai, New Delhi, and Trivandrum.**

When to take TOEFL?

You can take TOEFL all-round-the-year. The test is five-days-a-week (Monday through Friday).

How long is the score valid?

2 years

How to apply?

Online

The deadline to register online for a test is seven days before the test date.
For fastest and most convenient service, register online.
- A valid credit card is required (American Express®, Discover®, JCB®, MasterCard®, or Visa® card), or an electronic check (e-check) if you have a bank account in the United States or its territories.

By phone

You must call at least seven days before the test date. Valid credit card required.
Registration phone: 91-11-26511649.

By mail

Fill in all information on the *Registration Form* in the *Information and Registration Bulletin* available at the nearest USEFI center located in the US Consulate or you can download it from www.ets.org.

India
Prometric
160-A Senior Plaza, 3rd floor
Gautam Nagar
Yusuf Sarai: Behind Indian Oil Bldg.
New Delhi 110049 India
Courier Address:
Prometric
160-A, Senior Plaza, 3rd floor
Gautam Nagar
Yusuf Sarai: Behind Indian Oil Bldg.
New Delhi 110049 India
Registration phone: 91-11-26511649
Fax: 91-11-26529741

Web: www.prometricindia.com
Required at all test centers for all tests:
Valid passport **is mandatory.**
Secondary signature bearing identification, e.g., Driving License, Notarised identification.
Confirmation letter or number

APPLYING TO UNIVERSITIES IN THE US

HOW TO APPLY AND GET INTO A MASTERS PROGRAM?

The admission process

Careful planning is required to choose the schools that would fulfil your needs. Although the internet offers you enough information and opportunities to learn more about the programs and colleges that suit you the most, the following option wont hurt either:

1. Visit the US embassy and ask for educational information. They regularly organize seminars on educational options in the US. Their Library also carries a good selection of directories, guides, college catalogues. Additionally you can procure the GRE, GMAT, TOEFL and other Exam information booklet from them. Another good source of information is to attend US College fairs that are periodically conducted in major cities. Some of them even offer spot admission and scholarship.
2. Post-MBBS students pursuing graduate studies have an option of entering a masters program or a doctoral program, depending on the area of interest and future goals. Next step is choosing an institution. There are public and private institutions. Public institutions generally have lower tuition rates compared to private ones. Other than the financial difference, high quality programs exist in both.
3. Once you have procured enough information, develop a list based on which regions in the US you want to apply for. Look for a list of colleges in that area. Shortlist them (base your choice on geography, hospital experience opportunity, existence of scholarship, ranking, teaching assistant opportunities).
4. Compare the shortlisted programs and eliminate the ones that don't meet your criteria on financial costs or one that doesn't suit your professional needs.
5. Accessing university catalogues online is the most inexpensive and least time-consuming option. Download the application and list of required documents to be sent. The admission process varies among universities

and it is best to work with a shortlist of may be 10 places where you really would like to go. MOST IMPORTANT: Note down the deadlines for programs. Take into account delivery delays.

6. If information you seek is not available, contact the university via E-mail requesting a catalogue and application to be sent to your address.
7. You must start identifying institutions even before you take your admissions test. This way you can take the right exam and aim for the right scores and your resume may be reflective of how good a chance you have of gaining admission to a program. Ideally start this process right after your final year exams.
8. Most commonly required documents would be your undergraduate scores, admission test scores, a personal statement on your choice of vocation, financial support documents, application fee, at least 3 letters of recommendation. Prepare them early and file them separately.
9. Sending out applications can prove to be a costly affair. Identify a courier service agent and stick to one. This way you would get reliable service and also a rough idea of how long it will take for your documents to reach them. Some courier companies offer discount services to students and a flat rate envelope.
10. Then the waiting game begins. Be prepared to have telephone interviews at some places. It can be an opportunity for you to ask about the program.
11. Once you start getting your acceptance letters, then you can relax and choose where you want to go. Along with the acceptance letter you will get I-20 which is required for gaining a visa appointment at the consulate.
12. Don't panic if you feel you won't be able to schedule an appointment at the US embassy for the visa. You are eligible to seek a priority appointment 120 days before the program start date mentioned on the I-20. In case you feel your cutting date is too close, E-mail the US embassy requesting an appointment.

In case you feel the entire process is very time consuming, there are a wide number of professional consultancies who will guide you through the entire process from searching for universities to preparing you for the admissions tests and sending out applications. Be aware of fraudulent practices and choose a place that you can place your trust on. A good way would be to choose one with whom someone you personally know had a good experience with. Spend some time on researching the consultancy firm.

GETTING THE F1 VISA

Applying for the F1 visa

Once you have received your I-20 from your university, you could apply for your F1 visa days prior to the start date indicated in the I-20.

How to apply for the F1 visa?

Step 1: visit the website www.vfs-usa.co.in
This will give you an overview of the process involved and guide you through the procedure.

Step 2: Locate the nearest HDFC Bank designated to accept the VFS fee and Application fee.

The fees payable at HDFC Bank per passport are:

Visa Application Fee (MRV Fee): $100 in Indian Rupee equivalent at consular rate of exchange. Rupee amount at current rate of exchange (Rs. 46) is Rs 4,600/-.

This fee is payable in cash or by DD/HDFC Bank cheque favoring "US Embassy-Visa Fees". DDs issued by Cooperative Banks are not accepted.

VFS' Service Charge: Rs 281/- (inclusive of Service Tax @ 12% and Education Cess Tax @ 0.24%) This fee is payable in cash or by DD/HDFC Bank cheque favoring "HDFC Bank a/c VFS". DDs issued by Cooperative Banks are not accepted.

Step 3: The HDFC Fee receipt can be used for scheduling an interview appointment 1 year from the date of issue. Wait for 2 days before scheduling your appointment.

Step 4: Go to www.vfs-usa.co.in website and click on apply for non immigrant visa. You will need details from your passport, the HDFC Bank receipt and I-20 to fill the application.

Step 5: In case you need an early appointment, you could request for emergency visa appointment provided it's 120 days within the start date mentioned on the I-20. Another way would be to wait patiently in front of your computer, frequently checking for available dates by refreshing the page with the available date. Most often you will get a date convenient for you.

Step 6: In case you cannot find a date, you could contact the US embassy by Email requesting an appointment.

Step 7: Paying the SEVIS fee.

Online Payment

Go to www.fmjfee.com. You will need the SEVIS details on your I-20 to complete the documentation and pay the fee of 100 $ US. You can use Visa or Master Card, Debit or Credit card to pay this fee.

By Mail

You can download the I-901 form from http://www.ice.gov/sevis/I-901/index.htm
   http://www.ice.gov/doclib/sevis/pdf/I-901.pdf
   Fill out the form and attach check or money order for 100 $ US
   All checks and money orders must be made in US dollars and drawn on a bank located in the United States.
   Mail Form I-901 and the payment to:
   I-901 Student/Exchange Visitor Processing Fee
   PO Box 970020
   St. Louis, MO 63197-0020
   Or
   Courier Form I-901 and the payment to:
   I-901 Student/Exchange Visitor Processing Fee
   1005 Convention Plaza
   St. Louis, MO 63101
   Tip on courier service:
   DHL offers a discount flat rate for students. Check with other courier services for similar offers.

Preparing for the Visa Interview

1. Get at least 4 photographs of yourself according to the current specifications mentioned on your DS forms.
2. Print out all your confirmation letter and the DS forms for the visa interview appointment and proof of payment of SEVIS fee.
3. Your test scores.
4. Evidence of acceptance into an accredited US university or college program:
   I-20 issued by the university
   Acceptance letter
   Evidence of scholarship (if applicable)
5. Proof of previous educational experience (mark sheets from school and medical college).
6. Proof of previous and current employment (if applicable).

7. A copy of the course description and contents.
8. Evidence of binding ties to return to India on completion of your course.
   Covering letter from Chartered Accountant
   Property documents
   Marriage certificate if applicable
   Proof of any partnership in business
9. Sponsorship documents.
10. Bank statements and income tax returns.
11. Affidavit of support with relationship of the sponsor to you.

It would be best if you could find a folder with multiple compartments and place the above in them and label them and go through them before your actual interview.

Questions you must be prepared to answer:
- Why?
- Your course of study
- Your choice of university
- Choose to study now?
- How long do you intend to study in the US?
- What are your plans when you come back?
- What reasons do you have to come back here after your studies?
- How are you going to support yourself while you study?
- What does your father do?
- What is your annual income for your family?
- In what way will your course help you be a better physician?
- Why did you choose to do this following medicine?
- Have you considered doing residency in the US?
- You could practice these questions with someone and have a clear idea towards what your goals are. The best way to get through the interview is by being honest.

On the day of your appointment

Dress smartly and comfortably. Be relaxed. Make sure you have all the documents with you before you leave for the appointment. Start early. Do not be late for your appointment.

COMBINING A MASTERS PROGRAM AND USMLE

Tips on studying for the USMLE while on F1

1. Planning: Most courses should be flexible enough for you to be able to have

the weekend off as well as have another 2 days for you to concentrate on your Usmle preparation.
2. Answer the following questions for you to be able to prepare a timetable
   - What Steps are you planning to take, Step 1, Step2 CK or CS, Step 3?
   - How quick of a learner are you? How much time would you need for an ideal preparation for your exam?
   - What are your priorities? To finish your current program or aim to get into a residency as soon as possible and then continue to pursue your current course work?
   - Which year are you planning to match?
3. Common dilemmas:
4. Which Step to take first? Traditionally Step 1 basic sciences part takes up quite a lot of preparation when compared to the other Steps, partly due to the sheer volume of material to be assimilated as well as the time that has elapsed from the time we read our basic sciences till now when we have to go back and read concepts as well as keep focusing on the changing trends. Also behavioral science and some concepts in ethics would be quite new to master.

Step 2 CK: More clinically oriented study material. It's easier to prepare for, and ideal preparation time with an average of 8 sincere hours a day could be 4 months. If you have just finished your CRRI or your final year it would seem more practical to take this Step first.

Step 2 CS: Very clinical. Assuming that you are proficient in English, and what materials you would use for your preparation, you could take this exam in as little time as 3 weeks. Getting the dates for taking the exam and the place you want to take the exam might be a little tricky affair though. So plan ahead for this exam. Since the validity to schedule the exam is for a year, go ahead and apply for this exam if you are confident you will take this exam some time during this year. This will give you greater flexibility to take your exam at the date you want at your choosen location.

Step 3: This exam cannot be taken unless you are ECFMG certified. The advantage of taking Step 2 CK last truly shows here. If you follow the pattern of Step 1, 2 CS then CK, you will have your results within 4 weeks and get your ECFMG certificate around that time too if all your transcripts have been verified. It would take another maximum 3 weeks for you to apply and get the permit to take Step 3. It is possible to continue your preparation for Step 3 within that 7 week period, so you don't lose any time and you will be able to take the exam in 7 weeks with time enough for an ideal preparation. It also helps because Step 3 is an extended preparation from Step 2 materials with exam format changes.

Though it would not hurt to have a high score in Step 3, it's more of a formality in getting a H-1 B visa and a state license. Therefore, for many it might be a race against time to get this exam over within the last leg of journey towards getting into a residency program.

If you have taken Step 2 followed by Step 1 route then taking Step 3 is a little time-consuming. You might have to reread and refresh your clinical knowledge and preparation time could vary.

Once you have made your decision on which Step you want to take, the next Step is deciding what your priority is if you want to get into a residency program as early as you can or focus on your current course work and aim to complete it before embarking on your residency.

It is very possible to excel in your coursework and also study for your MLE's. Just that the time frame might vary based on your priorities.

Should I carry my books with me?

With the current baggage restrictions on the international traveler, it is quite difficult to choose what to take. I would definitely recommend taking your basic USMLE notes and personalized notes with you. A good rule of thumb while deciding is — am I going to use this book for reference? if yes then leave it back. It's likely your library at your school would be able to get you any textbook you want. If they don't have it, you can contact the inter-library loan dept at the library and they would be able to get it for you within a week or two. The Library reference desk would be able to answer any query you might have.

But be aware that making copies would prove to be expensive and tedious if it involves more pages as in almost all places you would need to make copies yourself. Also there is strict copyright rules. It's better to make full use of the library and the internet whenever possible. As a student you will enjoy the privilege of free internet access at your school.

How can I find a study partner?

If you are enrolled at university with a med school attached, then it's very simple. Look for flyers looking for a study partner or print some that you are looking for a study partner and give your contact number and put them on the allocated notice boards. If your university does not have a med school attached then you could find a med school nearest to you and do the same. In case you can't find one, the next best option is to join a forum like www.prep4usmle.com and follow-up the happenings on the forum and put a note looking for a study partner in your area or find an online study partner. Being in the US as a first timer with little or no friends can sometimes be lonely and here is a possibility of developing low feelings that can be detrimental to your preparation. Having a study partner can allay some of these feelings and you will not feel you are alone in this big, big world.

Tips if you want to complete your Steps as early as possible:

1. Take the minimum course requirements–for most university programs at graduate level would be 3 courses or 9 hours of classes.
2. Schedule your classes in successive days of the week or all on the same day. This way you would not have to waste time on travel and can stay focused on studying.
3. Most students would prefer to take an on-campus job to aid financially. If you can't avoid it, contact your human resources department at your school and look for jobs at the library or computer labs where work is sedentary and won't tire you out and may even give you time to study and access internet.
4. If you have finished your first semester and you feel you would rather come back home to prepare, it's possible to contact your international students advisor for a semester break. This way you can come to India and take the exams here (only Step1 and Step 2 CK) and have a new I-20 issued when you are ready to go back. It might not be very flexible as you have to enroll for a semester and wait for the semester to begin. Good planning is absolutely essential.
5. Another alternative is for you when you have completed your first semester: To transfer to KAPLAN which has centers in all major cities across the US for your preparation. That would still give you student status and in case you need to be there for an Observership or externship. This way you will be focused on your USMLE preparation completely. The drawback here is you won't be working towards an additional degree. Again get your priorities straight.
6. Summer semester is optional and that would be the best time to remain in the US and take exams. May thru July would be totally class free if you decide not to take any courses. If you had done your reading during the spring semester you can focus on working our questions and online Q banks and take the exam in this period. Winter breaks and spring breaks are too short of time though they can be ideal times for you to take Step 2 CS.

[11] Other Routes of Entering the United States

Muralikrishna G

1. RESEARCH AND H1 RESEARCH VISAS

Another commonly used route to enter the United States:
- The university must sponsor a J1 visa for you to enter the United States or a H1 visa for which the University has to pay about $ 3000-4000 to sponsor the visa for you.
- It can be basic science (bench research) or clinical science research.
- In basic science research, the job is usually a post-doctoral research fellow position in which one works in a designated laboratory under a research supervisor on a research project.
- In clinical research, one is usually employed as a Clinical Research Assistant (CRA) in research projects that may be ongoing in the university.
- Though theoretically anybody can apply for a research position in a US university with their CV from India, it does not work.
- The best chance is to have some personal contact in any university who can themselves or through their contacts get you the job as a post-doctoral fellow.
- It is usually a paid job (approx. $ 30,000 per year but varies widely) but could be unpaid too.
- The research experience in a US university considerably strengthens your residency application in terms of your interest in research, commitment to academics, knowledge of the US research environment, etc.
- This is the ideal situation in basic or clinical research: Work in a top-notch University Hospital (read Harvard or Johns Hopkins) from six months to a

year under a well known researcher, get a few publications in peer reviewed journals, present in an American or International Conference, in the field that you are applying for residency. If you can get all these factors together, you can get into competitive specialties and competitive programs.
- The obvious problem in a J1 research visa is that you can change only to a H1 clinical visa, a process that involves a lot of paperwork and takes about six months time.
- The problem with the H1 research visa is that it reduces the validity period of your visa. If you stay on a H1 research visa for 6 months or a year, then the time left on your H1 visa to do your residency and fellowship is reduced. The total duration of a H1 visa is six years, with a possible extension of one year. If you do research on a H1 visa for a year, and then Internal Medicine residency for three years, you would only have two years to complete your fellowship, whereas fellowships such as Cardiology and Gastroenterology are three years each. Then, in that case, one has to do a job after residency to get a Green Card before pursuing fellowship.

GREEN CARD

If you have parents or brothers/sisters living in the United States, they can sponsor a Green card for you. A Green card significantly increases your chances of getting more interviews, especially in competitive specialties and competitive programs.

F2/J2/H4 DEPENDENTS

If one gets married to someone who is in the United States as a student (F1 visa), then one goes on a F2 dependent visa. A J1 and H1 visa holder's spouse gets a J2 and an H4 dependent visa in view of their marriage.

MARRIAGE

A common route, especially in India to somehow enter the United States. These marriages may again be by choice or by chance. In the end, one gets a hassle free entry to the United States and the advantage of being considered for competitive programs and competitive specialties because of the visa status.

The above was a short introduction to the other routes of entering the United States. A detailed discussion about each of these topics is outside the scope of the book. The reader is advised to make use of the Internet and personal contacts to gather more information.

Section Four
Adding Weight to Your Application

12
Research Before Residency
Varun Agarwal

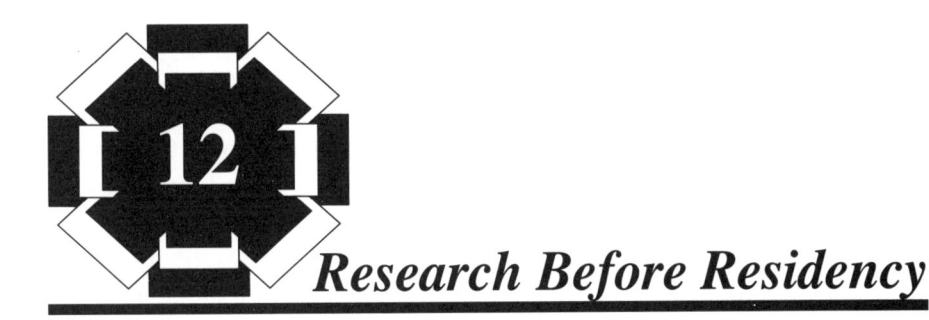

Now that medicine is rapidly moving towards evidence-based approach, it is vital to develop the ability to read and analyze research articles. One way to truly appreciate the nature of a research study and its implications is to involve oneself in research projects.

Having a research experience goes a long way to strengthen your application. There are many kinds of research projects—basic science, clinical, case report, etc. Research experience shows the residency programs that you took the pain and effort to acquaint yourself with the research terminology and that you know some of the basic biostatistical terms and how they are used to understand a research study.

Whether you want to do basic science research or clinical research is entirely a personal choice based on your previous experience and level of training. Basic science research needs much more time to get results and requires one to have a more thorough training in cell and molecular biology and lab research methodology. Big shot university based programs love to take in applicants with such a kind of research background as they are convinced that such applicants can contribute greatly to their programs by developing more research projects and getting research grants. An example would be "To determine how p38 MAPK causes insulin resistance in type 2 diabetic patients". Another way how basic science research helps is if you want to later on get into more competitive fellowships like cardiology and GI.

Not to say that clinical research is not equally important. Clinical research studies are usually shorter, can be completed faster and does not really require lots of specialized study. All residency programs however big or small appreciate clinical research. It appeals to a much wider audience. An example would be

"To determine whether intensive insulin therapy leads to a much greater lowering of Hb (A1c) (Allright this is a landslide study, but just to give you an example). Another interesting thing about clinical research is that a study can be created with many ways to look at it—for example the above study can be used to show your interest in either internal medicine, or endocrinology, or public health.

So the bottomline is that having a research experience gives an extra edge to your application. This will prove very useful especially when the competition is increasing.

The most ideal situation would be to involve yourself in a research project, complete it, send it to a conference for acceptance, presentation either oral or poster and lastly publish an article in a journal. As I said this is the most 'ideal' situation. You could also write in your application that you are working on the project and by the time you are called for interview show them your work or even the abstract if it's done.

The type of research you involve yourself in also makes some difference. Clinical research study carries much more weightage than say a case report.

For an IMG, it is best to get yourself into a research project in the US itself. This would allow you better chances for acceptance into national conferences. The credibility of your work will not be questioned, or can be evaluated if desired. Also you can get a letter of recommendation from your mentor.

University programs have lots of research projects going on at all times. So that's the best place to start in. Get in touch with a university program or a medical school. Each university's website gives in detail the nature of research work being carried out at their department. Find a topic that interests you and get in touch with the research mentor. Personal contacts can help very much. While doing so, do tell them about your prior research experiences if any, tell them about your basic computer skills and most importantly why you are interested in their research. It's best to be truthful and let them know that you are applying for a residency program and your long term goals.

Once you do that, based on how you approach, you might get a positive or a negative response. Do not be discouraged and keep trying and trying. If positive, set-up an appointment to meet the research mentor in person. Be professional in your approach. As an IMG, one of the important things to keep in mind is that your involvement, as many mentors like it to be, is purely voluntary. Of course there are also paid positions that might even offer you visa to work at their place with a salary. Do keep in mind that your aim out here is to get research experience and a letter of recommendation rather than make money. As I said, since it's a voluntary position, it's your job to convince the mentor about your commitment and that you will be definitely completing the research project at hand. Make sure you know how many hours and how many months you can spend especially if you are in the middle of taking the USMLE Steps. Make a schedule beforehand if possible. And do mention the type of visa you are in.

Again you will be judged on your professionalism, your honesty, your willingness to complete the project that will go in your favor. Once you get the nod, congratulations, you have now embarked yourself on a winning strategy that will take you much higher into a much better residency program.

Summer is the best time to get involved in research projects (April, May). Classes for medical students are typically shut down during this time and the professors have more time to spend on research. Starting in summer will also give you ample time to make a significant contribution by September when you actually start applying. And by the time of interviews in November, you would have known where exactly your research is headed and can talk about it sufficiently and confidently during the residency interviews.

Having said that, do keep in touch with your mentor and the other research faculty at least till the time of the match. Do not exit leaving a bad taste in the mouth of the mentor. That is, never leave the project midway or hanging in the middle just because you got a position or for any other reason. This is highly unprofessional of a physician.

Getting to know the other research faculty who are in touch with your mentor is very helpful to make contacts. Very often you will encounter big shots who will go a long way to help you in your quest for a residency program. Do make sure you can make a good and lasting impression on them.

Research meetings are usually held once a week. All the research faculties get together at this time and go over the progress of the research projects. This is the best time to show your work and interest. Do not be bogged down if they don't like your idea. Try to improvise on it and present again. Show your knowledge of the subject, your interest and how you can contribute best to completing it. You would have to go through research articles and learn what kind of work has been done in a certain field and what needs to be done. This will give you an idea of what your research project is going to involve. This takes a lot of time and lot of discussion but once you know what you are aiming for, you are in good shape.

Deciding who your mentor is going to be is an important issue of its own. Obviously working under someone who is well renowned in their field certainly carries a lot of weightage, but if they are so busy, they will not have enough time to be available to you when you need their input. Worse, they might not even get to know you sufficiently well to write a strong recommendation. So make sure you choose your mentor wisely—they need to know you, your idea, your work ethic well enough to appreciate all your work. And you would not want to work under someone who is short-tempered or malignant.

Once you have a research idea on hand, the next step obviously is to implement it. Firstly most of the programs have an online learning module on human subject research that every researcher involved with human subjects needs to take (www.citiprogram.org). It's free and can be done easily.

The next thing would be to submit your idea to a Human Investigation committee at the place where you plan to do the research. Your mentor helps with most of that work so you don't need to get stressed on that. It's basically that you are presenting your research idea to a committee to show that your research is ethical and will not harm patients (or minimally) in any way. They usually accept it and ask you to go ahead with your project.

The next step is to work on the intricate details on how you plan to do your project. If it requires chart review, you would need to make the database for easy entry. If it requires handing patient questionnaires, you need to work on that. This is where it takes the maximum time. Planning ahead will save you a lot of trouble later on. Your mentor will help you in deciding how best to approach your research idea.

After the methodology has been formulated, the next step is data collection. Studies involving chart review, lab studies don't require patient contact. Make sure you have enough patients so that the power of the study is adequate and the data is not skewed. If patient contact is required, as in patient questionnaires or taking interviews, you have to prepare a HIPAA consent form. This basically tells the patient that patient data will not be discussed with anyone except the researchers mentioned on that form. You need to explain to the patient what the study is about, why it needs to be done, how it can help others, how many visits would be required and how the patient can contribute to it. Spell out everything to the patient and answer any questions they have. You need to get the patients' consent in doing so and hand them a copy so that they can withdraw from the study if required at a later time. Having a financial compensation helps at times, but sometimes you may not be lucky and must earn patients' trust and goodwill in you to help out with your 'career'.

At this time more and more helping hands will let you collect data much faster. The boring part is to enter all the data into a database like MS Access. Make sure you have ways to doublecheck the data you are entering. Next comes data analysis. Most of us are not aware of softwares like SPSS, SAS that perform statistical analysis. For doing basic statistical calculations like creating a table, calculating mean, p value, statistical significance, it can be interesting to learn these basic concepts. For further analysis like regression, it's better to get professional help from a biostatistician.

As with any research study, it's best if your p value is significant. Your mentor will help you out with that. Sometimes it pays to explore and work out different ways of looking data to get statistical significance or even a linear trend in data.

A quick note about case reports, since it's a case vignette describing something interesting you saw in a patient, you don't have to go through all the above data analyses.

Now that all data have been collected and analyzed and you got your results, it's time to tell the world about your research. Discuss submitting your research to a national (or international) conference with your mentor. This would involve, at first, writing an abstract and submitting it to the review committee of that conference for acceptance.

Writing an abstract is an art of its own. Every conference has its own requirements like word limit, font size and stick strictly to that. Abstracts have different parts to it—introduction, reason why you did the study, what the study involved, results, discussion and conclusion. All these aspects have to be written clearly without any ambiguity in your abstract. You need to be concise, to the point but still explain the whole picture to your audience.

Submitting to national conferences is always preferable—it might be difficult to get in as the competition might be stiff, but once your abstract is accepted, the value of your study shoots up exponentially. Keep in mind that many conferences do not allow you to present a study if it had been presented in any other conference. So do discuss with your mentor if your study is worth sending to a national conference or a local meeting.

The best method of presentation is oral. This is always preferred and tough to get in. This involves explaining to an audience your study and its outcome (in powerpoint slides) and answering the questions from the audience. You need not get scared, as your mentor would be sitting next to you (hopefully) to help you out with sticky situations. But do realize that oral presentation requires a lot of clear thinking and understanding.

The next best method is poster presentation. You would have to create a poster and give a short summary of your study to people who seem interested in your study. If it's a great poster, you even get prize for that. So don't get bogged down if your study does not get accepted for oral presentation.

The not so best way to present is just publication of your abstract in the conferences journal. But nevertheless you have a reference to write in your CV whenever required.

While you are doing all this, do make sure you share your progress on your research study with the programs where you interviewed. Besides giving an excuse for you to write to the program and keeping them on the top of their head, they will appreciate your hard work and effort and look upon you very favorably.

After all this has been done and if you still have a lot of time on hand, the next best thing would be to write-up your study as a research article in a journal. This is a whole different topic of its own and beyond the reach of this book. By this time your mentor has full faith in your effort and abilities and will be more than willing to help you out with writing it up.

The bottomline is that getting yourself involved in a research project is a different and interesting experience of it's own. Even if it doesn't help you in your residency, it's always good to keep an open mind and think of research ideas as you go ahead in your career. It would also help you better and more critically read journal articles as you would now know how the author would have designed and carried out the whole research study.

Another thing to keep in mind is that, be a bit cautious about what you tell the program director during the interview. If you have done a lot of basic science research and tell the PD of a community hospital with no basic science research labs that you want to explore cell and molecular biology, you will never be taken in that program (of course you would have much better interview calls). And when you go to a big university program, steer the talk towards your research study and how much you worked for it, how you learned, how it helped you in your career and so forth. So tailor your mode of presentation depending on whom you are interviewing with.

Research experience does help a lot to get into a program as I explained above. It will even help you in your search for a fellowship as it establishes your interest in research. So do take it seriously and grab every opportunity that you can get research experience.

United States Clinical Experience (USCE)

Muralikrishna G

INTRODUCTION

United States Clinical Experience (USCE) has emerged as an important factor in the residency application process, especially in the last few years. In this chapter, let us discuss the issue of US Clinical Experience.

ARE YOU A MEDICAL STUDENT OR A GRADUATE?

The fundamental question before we start this chapter is whether you are a medical student or a medical graduate. If one is a medical student, then one usually does a clinical elective in a US University during third/fourth year and internship. If one is a medical graduate, then one applies for an Observership/Externship and does the same on the visa that they entered the United States on.

MEDICAL GRADUATE

HOW TO GET AN OBSERVERSHIP?

How to find an observership?

1. Identify your contacts... however remote and far-fetched they may be... anybody in the Health care sector from secretaries to physician assistants... and request them.... they will know somebody in turn... presidents, private practitioners, faculty, even Program Directors sometimes... that is luck... but

this is the surest way of getting into a hospital... personal contact... many of you would have realized how much personal contacts matter in the US... a combination of SKILL and CONTACTS is quintessential in any career in the US.... most importantly in the US...
2. Finding out places close to your residence: The place where you stay... even your relatives or landlords may know Doctors in a Hospital nearby... who can get a foot in the door for you... then it is up to you... to meet the PD or any other important person and convince him that you need the Observership...
3. Finding out where Observerships are offered in the US: A lot of Observerships are paid these days... and there is intense competition for the paid Observerships too...

GO MEET THEM

Find out application requirements, availability here, for this option, you have to compromise... move to a new city... find accommodation, food, etc... Only if you can put in that effort... can you reap benefits...
4. YOUR CV.... if your CV is good enough, you can get an Observership far easily. Because PD s want you as a resident... they can impress you when you come as an observer... in the US... Everything is a business... even resident selection... so PD will think miles ahead of you.

WHAT TO DO DURING THE OBSERVERSHIP?

I've summarized what I've learnt over the last two months applying for Observerships...

This message is intended for those doing an Observership or planning to do one...
1. First few days, orientation, immunization tests, HIPPA, confidentiality agreement and ID card.
2. I had meeting with PD, I wanted detailed schedule, rotations in various departments, opportunity to do H/O and physicals both in clinics and wards, clinical discussion, and presentation.
3. The faculty were wonderful enough to let me see patients in the clinic even before they saw them individually... the best thing that could ever happen... then they saw each patient with me... and let me write patient notes... interpret ECGs... laboratory data...
4. In the wards.... less active... esp coz of nurses... but again I could spend quality time with patients... sometimes upto an hour.... to take detailed history and physical... and then present and discuss patients during morning report...

5. Learnt a little of medical coding, dictation and insurance issues
6. Pushed PD for presentation... finally last week, I made presentation on topic given by PD, "Anti-depressants in depression" BASED ON RECENT ARTICLE IN BMJ... went on so well... faculty were very impressed...
7. Next week... presentation in grand rounds... presentation of a case of rhabdomyosarcoma seen by a pediatrician recently...
8. Also given me research project of working on Troponin I in myocardial infarction... 4 week study... retrospective.... access to medical records of hospital... something most faculty don't get... so I learnt how the records worked... how they are archived and filed... etc.

HOW TO GET LETTERS OF RECOMMENDATION?

- Identify faculty who can give letters of recommendation.
- Work closely with those faculty.
- Participate actively in the academic meetings of the hospital- morning report, noon conference, journal club and grand rounds.
- Perform clinical research under faculty and try to present cases in the morning report, noon conference and grand rounds.
- After you are confident that you can get a good letter of recommendation, write a requisition letter and give it to the letter writers and ask them if they know you well enough to write a strong letter of recommendation. Then, whether you get the letter or not and how strong it is depends on how well you have done during the Observership.
- *Ideal letter:* From a Program Director/Chair or attending of a University Hospital with a residency program where you worked alongside the residents, with hands-on clinical experience, performed research and did clinical presentations and the LOR talks specifically about your strengths and strongly recommends you for a residency program.

DOING RESEARCH AND PRESENTATIONS

During the Observership, one can do clinical presentation during the morning report based on an interesting patient you may have seen in the last few weeks, especially something that can be a useful educational tool for residents. You can request the faculty for a presentation during the noon conference where you can either discuss a recent article in a medical journal or give a talk on a common disease process or public health problem.

WHICH PLACES OFFER OBSERVERSHIPS?

There are numerous hospitals that offer Observerships in the US as an official program...

Hospitals providing Observership or externship in the US: Columbia University (Med)

Contact person is Mr. Leon Bynum 212-305-1642

Wilson Memorial Regional Medical Center (Med)
James R. Fowler, Jr. 607-763-6392
James_Fowler@uhs.org
www.uhs.net/meded

Cooper Health System (Med)

Mount Sinai Medical System (Med)
marianna.vougioukas@mssm.edu

Griffin Hospital (Med)
USF Dept. of Internal Medicine
Cheryl Beckler (813-974-4881 or cbeckler@hsc.usf.edu). She schedules all the observerships in the Department of Internal Medicine (no externships offered).

Orlando Regional health care (Med)
You must have proof of insurance when you apply for clerkship.
You could go into www.orhs.org and print out the clerkship application.
Aracelis Febo
Residency Coordinator
Aracelis.Febo@orhs.org

University of Miami (Med)
Andrea Ruiz
University of Miami (R-760)
Department of Medicine
Dominon Towers, Suite 807D
PO Box 016760
Miami, FL 33101
(305) 243-8273 Office
(305) 243-5819 Fax

Tufts Medical School (Med)
VGelardi@tufts-nemc.org

Weill Medical College of Cornell University (Surgery)
Myndie Friedman
Program Administrator
Weill Medical College of Cornell University
Dept. of Surgery
212-746-6591 Phone
212-746-8802 Fax

Carolinas Medical Center (Surgery)
UNC Chapel Hill the contact person
Leanne Shook. Her number is 919-962-8338

UVM College of Medicine/Fletcher Mount Sinai (Surgery)
(802) 847-2566 - Fax (802) 847-9528

VCUHS-MCV Campus (Surgery)
Externships are handled by their School of Medicine. Their # is 804-828-9784. If you are interested in an observership, you will need to contact the specific division of surgery you are interested in to inquire. Please visit the website at www.surgery.vcu.edu for a list of surgery divisions and contact information.
Ms. Fonda Health
General Surgery Residency Coordinator
VCUHS - MCV Campus
PO Box 980135
Richmond, VA 23298
(804) 828-2755 Phone
(804) 828-5595 Fax
FHEATH@VCU.EDU

Flecher Allen Health Care (Surgery)
Diantha Langmaid
Surgery Resident Coordinator
UVM College of Medicine/Fletcher Allen Health Care
(802) 847-2566 - Fax (802) 847-9528

Aultman Hospital (GYN)
Beth Schmaltz
OB/GYN Residency and Clerkship Coordinator
Aultman Hospital
OB/GYN Department

2600 Sixth Street SW
Canton OH 44710
(330) 363-6214 Phone
(330) 363-5228 Fax

MEDICAL STUDENT

As a medical student, the pros of doing an elective are tremendous.
1. You can spend 1-2 months in the US doing electives/rotations in the specialty you will be applying for a few years from then.
2. You will almost surely get the visa to enter the United States.
3. You will get hands-on clinical experience of working with patients and assisting in clinical procedures.
4. You can get strong letters of recommendation since you are being judged alongside fellow medical students only.
5. You will have a tremendous advantage when you apply for residency over those who have not done electives.

HOW TO GET AN ELECTIVE?

The American Association of Medical Colleges (AAMC) offers a link to all available clinical electives in the US.

The Extramural Electives Compendium (EEC) contains essential information for medical students about elective opportunities at Liaison Committee on Medical Education (LCME) accredited medical schools in the United States and Canada.

This information is used by the US and Canadian medical students, usually during the third and fourth years of their medical education, in planning and revising their academic schedules. It is also used by international medical students seeking enrollment in elective programs at the US and Canadian medical schools.

This information includes

- The name, address, telephone and fax number, and e-mail address of the appropriate contact person at each medical school.
- When applicable, the Web address(es) for the medical school and for related materials (e.g., curriculum brochures, application materials).
- The earliest date application materials are accepted.
- The earliest date that accepted visiting students can be assigned to available electives.

- The maximum number of weeks a visiting student can enroll in electives at the medical school.
- The application, tuition, and other fees charged to the visiting student.
- The amount of malpractice insurance required of each visiting student and the cost of the school-sponsored malpractice insurance program, when available.
- Any other school requirements for enrollment in electives.

Each school annually prepares a separate curriculum document listing electives available at that institution. The document is sent to all other medical schools (or the information is published on the school's Web site) to provide all available elective information to medical students planning on elective courses at those schools.

One usually has to send a set of documents, including CV and USMLE Step 1 scores, following which the University will decide if they want to take you in for the elective, then you get the visa to travel to the US, make all the necessary travel arrangements, spend 1-2 months in the US and come back. Some electives are paid and most require malpractice insurance. Another factor to consider is the cost involved, which may be anywhere from 2-3 lakhs.

WHAT TO DO DURING THE ELECTIVE? HOW TO GET LETTERS OF RECOMMENDATIONS?

The same issues that apply to Observerships, discussed above, apply here.

WHICH PLACES OFFER ELECTIVES?

http://www.aamc.org/students/medstudents/electives/start.htm
http://services.aamc.org/eec/student.cfm

REFERENCES

http://www.aippg.net/forum/viewtopic.php?t=24225
http://www.imgfriendlylist.com
http://www.essentialmedicine.net/imgessential/observershipsinus_Med1.php

Section Five
The Process of Getting into a US Residency

14

Choosing A Specialty

Nirav Mamdani

INTRODUCTION

The choice of specialty, as an International Medical Graduate, is limited, far more difficult and by and large dictated by the number and nature of positions not preferred by American Medical Graduates.

Broadly speaking, there are two kinds of specialties:
- Competitive
- Non-competitive

Two kinds of programs:
- Competitive
- Non-competitive

A majority of IMGs get into the non-competitive programs in the non-competitive specialties. The idea of this book is to increase your chances of getting into better programs in competitive specialties.

WHAT SPECIALTIES ARE AVAILABLE?

- Anesthesiology
- Child Neurology (Neurology)
- Dermatology
- Emergency Medicine
- Family Medicine
- Internal Medicine
- Internal Medicine/Emergency Medicine
- Internal Medicine/Family Practice

118 Acing the USMLE and the Match

- Internal Medicine/Pediatrics
- Internal Medicine/Physical Medicine and Rehabilitation
- Internal Medicine/Psychiatry
- Neurology
- Neurological Surgery
- Nuclear Medicine
- Obstetrics and Gynecology
- Orthopaedic Surgery
- Otolaryngology
- Pathology–Anatomic and Clinical
- Pediatrics
- Pediatrics Dermatology
- Pediatrics/Emergency Medicine
- Pediatrics/Physical Medicine and Rehabilitation
- Pediatrics/Psychiatry/Child and Adolescent Psychiatry
- Physical Medicine and Rehabilitation
- Plastic Surgery
- Psychiatry
- Psychiatry/Family Practice
- Psychiatry/Neurology
- Radiation Oncology
- Radiology–Diagnostic
- Surgery–General
- Transitional Year
- Urology

HOW DO I CHOOSE A MEDICAL SPECIALTY AS AN IMG?

Which Specialty?

Bottomline: Go for the specialty that you are interested in.

You do not want to get stuck with something that you do not LIKE to do.

At the same time, remember that some specialties are more competitive than others.

In general, primary care residencies like Categorical (rather than Preliminary) internal medicine, pediatrics, obstetrics and gyn, family medicine, psychiatry and neurology are relatively easy to get.

Categorical General surgery (rather than Prelim Surgery), anesthesia are more competitive than primary care specialties, but still there are quite a good number of IMGs in them.

Radiology, dermatology, ENT, ophthalmology, orthopedics and emergency medicine are very difficult residencies to get. This is true not only for IMGs but also for AMGs.

Some specialties like Nuclear Medicine and Genetics are unexplored and may not necessarily be difficult to get into.

In general, surgical specialties are more difficult than medical specialties. This is mainly due to the fact that there is no set standard to assess the surgical skills of IMGs. (as opposed to medical specialties, where standardized exams may help assess knowledge base of candidates). This is the main reason why most IMGs have to do either prelim year or have US experience in some other form prior to getting accepted in any surgical specialties.

For any specialty, university programs are more difficult to get in than community programs. Ivy league programs (Harvard, Stanford, Johns Hopkins, Mayo, etc.) are extremely difficult to get in.

Most programs prefer AMGs over IMGs with similar credentials; however, if an IMG has clearly superior credentials, the program will definitely rank him/her higher than other candidates.

How to select a specialty?

Following factors need to be considered:
1. *You MUST like to work in that specialty!* You cannot commit yourself to something that you don't like.
2. *Consider lifestyle issues:* Some specialties are more demanding in terms of work hours than others. For example, endocrinology or rheumatology has much softer work hours than cardiology or orthopedics. In many specialties you can tailor your work hours. One good example is internal medicine: after internal medicine you can either decide to work only during 9-5 in outpatient setup or you can elect to work as hospitalist which may involve night time work hours.
3. *Consider the pay scales:* In general you can easily make more money than you will need for decent living; no matter which specialty you go to. Also remember that the amount of money you make is generally proportional to the amount of work you do and amount of responsibilities you have. Overall, surgical specialties pay more than medical specialties. You can get most recent average salaries in various specialties on website www.salary.com. Remember that these are average numbers and there are extreme outliers on either side of mean.
4. *Consider fellowship options:* If you are not very sure of your final choice, consider a residency that keeps various fellowship options open. For example,

after internal medicine you can either go to more intense and demanding fellowships like cardiology or nephrology or go to more laid-back fellowships like endocrine and rheumatology.

The chapter on different specialties, later in the book, will throw more light on the different options available to IMGs on choosing a specialty.

REFERENCES

http://services.aamc.org/eras/erasstats
http://www.aamc.org/audienceeras.htm

[15]

J1 Vs H-1B—The Million Dollar Question

Nirav Mamdani

INTRODUCTION

If you do not have a Green card or US citizenship, you have to do your residency on a J1 or an H-1B visa. Which visa to choose is definitely a difficult decision with pros and cons on either side of the divide. This chapter is written with the purpose of assisting you with the decision-making process.

THE H1 VISA

Visa issues related to H1 visa

1. A very good number and mixture (meaning big universities to small community) programs sponsor H1 visa. Those programs who do not sponsor H1 visa do it as they do not know what it is and how easy it is to do it. Legally it is never a big deal. Only a handful of programs really ever had legal issues; and that too due to their laxities and now they do not sponsor H1 visa any more. I have seen many times, even programs that say they will offer only J1 visa eventually sponsor H1 visa after the match! (all you have to do is to let them know that process is actually simpler than J1 visa!). Programs that do not sponsor H1 visa are not BETTER programs. Exception to this are programs that get NIH funding to partially sponsor their residency/fellowship and by law it cannot be utilized for H1 visa candidates. There are only a handful of programs that have this genuine legal problem with H1 visa.

2. The biggest advantage of H1 visa is that at the end of residency/fellowship you have much better chance of a better employment opportunity and flexibility compared to J1 visa.
   a. I will explain this by examples: at the end of residency many of my colleagues who were going for jobs/green cards were offered job at institutions like Cleveland clinic, William Beaumont hospital, etc. who will sponsor their green card. (These are not extraordinary candidates). I don't think you can get J waiver at such top notch places! they are getting a great start to their job career; and that too only for the duration of green card processing (the GC processing is detailed below); after that they may stay there or do something else. You do not have that liberty with J1 visa.
   b. With J1 visa you will first have to do at least three years of waiver (only a few people are lucky to get it at a decent place). Waiver has to be in primary care track and so if you are looking for waiver after fellowship it is actually more difficult to get and most of the time you will end up doing primary care for the entire duration of waiver even if you are actually a qualified sub-specialist. Then you start with the same H1 visa process (as mentioned under a) unless you are at a VA hospital where you can work for another two years and file for Green card under NIW category... so at least 5 years of working in underserved area and may be more.

Green card processing

Green card processing time: This is currently greatly different for people who are Born in India or China Vs. people who are not born in India or China.
   a. For people not born in India or China: Expected duration of entire GC processing is 1-2 years.
      i. It takes 2-4 months for labor certification now known as PERM processing, after which they can file I 140 and I 485 together. At the same time they can file for EAD and Advance parole (AP- also known as travel document). EAD and AP come in about 3 months. At this point you can travel in and out of the US freely without any visa requirements.
      ii. Then another 6-8 months for I 140 and once I 140 is approved you can change employers on portability while awaiting I 485 which takes variable time from 6 months to 2 years.
   d. For people born in India or China: Expected duration of GC processing is about 5-7 years (because of issue of "retrogression")
      i. It takes 2-4 months for labor certification now known as PERM processing, after which they can only file I 140 and not I 485 (until about another five years or so due to retrogression). At this they cannot file for EAD and

J1 Vs H-1B—The Million Dollar Question

Advance parole. And so it is advisable to be on H1 visa during this period to be able to travel outside the US for this entire duration. That means you should file for GC at least before the end of fifth year on H1 visa.

ii. In about 6-8 months I 140 gets approved and then you can change employers on portability while awaiting I 485 dates to become current (which currently takes about five years or so as mentioned above), then you can file for I 485 which will be approved in another 6 months to two years.

WHAT AFTER H1 VISA?

Another burning question is, what do you do after six years on H1 visa? There are a lot of options!!

a. *Option 1:* If you are in a three year fellowship program, and if you find an employer 15-18 months in advance to file for green card (which is not difficult at all) then you can get your labor certification done and I 140 filed (not approved) before the beginning of last year of fellowship; then you can keep extending your H1 visa till GC gets approved totally and again same rules apply for the process I described above.

b. *Option 2:* If you have a lot of publications, you can file for EB1 category green card on you own during fellowship and if that gets approved, Bingo..! you got it. Not for everyone but many people do meet the criteria (there are ten criteria and you should meet three of them, they are listed on www.uscis.gov).

c. *Option 3:* Let's talk about the worst case scenario: you get employer just close to the end of your fellowship (and trust me, you will get that!! even in internal medicine people get 4-5 local employers hunting behind them) you still can file for green card and start working, all you cannot do is; you cannot extend your H1 visa and so you cannot travel outside the US till you get Advance Parole (which comes in about a year for people not born in India or China and about 5-6 years for people born in India or China) and then you can travel freely. During this entire period you are not on any status; just pending green card.

d. *Option 4:* "Reset the H1 visa clock". All you have to do is to stay out of the US for one year (it does not matter where you go, you may go to your home country, or any other country doing job or just go for world tour!!) and you get another six years on your H1 visa!!

Getting fellowship on H1 visa: It is not impossible or even more difficult to get fellowship on H1 visa. I can tell my own experience: out of 170 cardiology programs in the country 90 sponsors H1 visa and similar number sponsors J1 visa!! If you are a good candidate, visa is not an issue. Even the programs that do not sponsor H1 visa for internal medicine will sponsor H1 visa for fellowship!! (Example, SUNY Syracuse and there are quite a few on this list).

J1 Vs H1 VISA

Getting visa stamped: In general both H1 and J1 visa are not difficult to get stamped. H1 visa is considered a "dual intention visa" and that's why it cannot be rejected on the basis of "intending immigrant clause" (section 214B). J1 visa can be rejected with that section. Luckily it is uncommon to have any issues at all with stamping of either visa. J1 visa needs to be renewed every year, while H1 visa is usually for 3 years at a time.

Expense related to the visa: On an average it costs about $2500 to $4000 for H1 visa processing (depending on attorney fees). Cost for J1 visa is about $1000 (you do not need attorney for this). Processing time can be somewhat shorter with H1 visa with premium processing; but overall processing time is not too much different and usually not a problem at all.

Most of the time moonlighting is not allowed on J1 visa. You can do moonlighting on H1 visa (within institution). If you are on H1 visa, your dependent spouse (on H4 visa) cannot work unless he/she gets his/her own H1 visa. If you are on J1 visa, your dependent spouse (on J2 visa) can get an EAD and work.

Total duration on H1 visa is six years at a time (after which either you have to file GC or reset the clock with one year outside US) whereas you can have total seven years on J1 visa. (after which you have to do waiver or go back to your home country for two years).

16

The Nuts and Bolts of Residency Application

Archana Bhaskaran, Muralikrishna G

I. INTRODUCTION

After the lengthy process of taking the USMLE Steps, comes the most awaited and nerve-wracking experience of applying for the US residency. The residencies in the US start on July 1st of every year. The application process starts in June of the previous year. The match is the computerized process by which applicants are matched into different residencies in the United States. This chapter is discussed in a chronological order starting with June of the year before the match to July of the year when you can start residency. For example, if you want to start your residency in July 1st 2009, you must start the application process in June 2008. So the chapter on June of year preceding match refers to the June 2008 in case of the July 2009 residency start date.

If you have come this far, congratulation, you have won half the battle. The rest is background work (for the application process) and pure luck (for the match) with a little contribution from your personality (for the interviews).

TIMELINES AND DEADLINES

ERAS 2008 Applicant Timeline (www.aamc.org)

Date	Activity
Mid June 2007	ERAS 2007 Applicant Manuals will be available for PDF download by chapters or in its entirety.
Late June 2007	Schools may begin to generate and distribute My ERAS tokens to applicants.

126 Acing the USMLE and the Match

July 1, 2007	MyERAS Web site opens to applicants to begin working on their applications.
September 1, 2007	Applicants may begin applying to ACGME accredited programs
September 1, 2007	ACGME accredited programs may begin contacting the ERAS Post office to download application files.
November 1, 2007	MSPEs are released.
December 2007	Military Match
January 2008	Urology Match
February 2008	Osteopathic Match
March 2008	NRMP Match results will be available.
May 31, 2008	ERAS Post office will close to prepare for the 2008 season.

CHRONOLOGICAL TIME FRAME

- June of year preceding match
- July of year preceding match
- July of year preceding match
- Before August of year before match
- Before September 1st of year preceding match
- September 1st of year preceding match
- USMLE Step 3 exam
- NRMP Registration
- The Interview season: Nov/ Dec/ Jan of year preceding match
- Pre match
- Rank order list deadline
- Match week
- Post-match scramble

II. JUNE OF YEAR PRECEDING MATCH

Step 1 and 2 CK should have been cleared prior to June of the preceding year of MATCH.

III. JULY OF YEAR PRECEDING MATCH

Step 2 CS June, July of the preceding year. This clinical skills Exam can be taken only in the US and if this timeline is followed, your results will be ready when you apply on September 1st. Another advantage of taking Step 2 CS early is, you will be ECFMG certified by September 1st. ECFMG certificate is issued once the candidate clears USMLE Step 1, 2 CK and CS. It takes a maximum of one week to 10 days after the CS result to get the ECFMG certificate, provided Step 1 and 2 CK have been cleared. If you are ECFMG certified at the time of applying to the universities (programs) you have a definite advantage. This certificate is not a necessity to apply to the programs.

ERAS/ECFMG Token

It is generally issued in the 2nd week of July or earlier. It can be bought via OASIS (Online Application Status and Info System), the same OASIS that is used to track your USMLE score reports. It costs $75. Electronic Residency Application Services (ERAS) is the means by which you will apply to the programs. It is an online service where you file in your details and send in some documents (Post/Mail) like transcript, LOR, etc. The first step towards this is to buy the ERAS Token. Within a few days you will be issued an ERAS Token number using which you can register at "my eras" and obtain your (Association of American Medical Colleges) AAMC id. This AAMC id is what you will be using to log in to your online application at my eras. The "my eras" link can be clicked on from the eras website. With this AAMC id your my eras account is activated and you can start filling your application.

IV. BY AUGUST OF YEAR BEFORE MATCH

A. Observership

This has gained a lot of importance especially since the 2006 match. The focus has shifted from the USMLE scores to US Clinical Experience. This is covered in a different chapter but July, August is the right time to do an Observership. Do note that this early Observership has 2 advantages.

a. It can be mentioned in your application when you apply in September. Once you have submitted the application, changes cannot be made later, nor can it be updated except in the "My Profile" section which includes your contact details only.

b. You will also be able to get a Letter of Recommendations (LOR) for the Observership which can be sent to the ERAS (Electronic Residency Application Services) to include in your application. Of course, LOR can be sent much later too, after applying.

B. Reserach the Programs

There is no one particular website which gives you information about what the programs are looking for in a candidate. Therefore it is necessary to email each of them and ask their requirements. General information about the program can be obtained from www.freida.com including their web address and contact info.

Using this, email each of the programs you are interested in with the following questions.
a. Do they have any cut off for the USMLE scores below which they do not consider?
b. Any criteria regarding multiple attempts in any exam?
c. Criteria regarding how old a medical graduate you can afford to be to apply? Most universities favor recent graduates.
d. The most important question is—Do they accept foreign Medical Graduates?
e. Do they sponsor visas, and if so what visa? J1 visa is sponsored by ECFMG but the programs should be willing to accept a candidate with J1. However H1 visa can be sponsored only by the university.
f. Do they offer observerships? If you are interested in an observership do this research work a little earlier.

Do not forget to provide some personal information about yourself like your scores, etc.

Apart from mailing them, visit each website and browse "residents". One indicator of the friendliness of the program to International Medical Graduates is the number of Foreign Medical Graduates in the program. You can also view the opinion of the residents in the program at 'scutwork.com'.

C. How to Choose Programs Which give a Positive Reply:

This is individualized once you satisfy their criteria you have to shortlist them in the following manner.
a. *Specialty of interest.* Nowadays FMGS are being accepted in Psychiatry, Pediatrics, Internal Medicine, Surgery, Obstetrics and Gynecology, Pathology, Anesthesia. So you can shortlist based on your field of interest although the latter ones are more difficult to get.
b. *Geographic area:* Some people prefer the East Coast, others the southern states, etc. for varied personal reasons. Some prefer to stay in big cities rather than small towns. These help to narrow down the options.
c. *University vs Community Programs:* Most people lean towards one or the other. The basic differences between the 2 are university programs offer better opportunities for fellowship especially in competitive fields like Cardiology and Gastroenterology, whereas community programs offer a more relaxed life style. University programs absorb their residents into their

fellowship programs which is quite convenient. This is only a general view and there are a lot of exceptions. A classic exception is Cook County Hospital, Chicago, which is one of the most taxing programs with plenty of fellowship positions. A University Hospital also has more ongoing research projects which might interest you.

However the experience gathered as a resident is equivalent whether from a university or a community setup. In general it is good to apply to UH: CH in a 50:50 basis.

d. *How good your curriculum vitae is:* A person with an excellent CV stands a good chance of getting into top programs. By excellent CV, I mean those having US Clinical experience (hands-on), a few published papers, may be UK/European Clinical Experience, excellent USMLE scores and in addition to this being a Green Card holder or a US citizen. Don't worry if you do not have these. Most of us do not and still manage to get into good programs if not the top ones. In general, every candidate should apply to top programs ranging in number from 2–10. Who knows, you may be the lucky!

e. *How complete your application is:* This is a very important factor. You score over others if you are ECFMG certified at the time of your application. This is in contrast to a person who has cleared just one Step. In fact I would rate a candidate with lower scores but a more complete application higher than better scores but incomplete application. If you are very particular about getting into a good program and if your application is incomplete then wait and apply for the following match. If you are not very particular then apply to the less competitive programs and you will be rewarded with results.

f. *Inside information:* This is the most important of all that have been listed. The information gathered and stratified from the programs in reply to your mail on the criteria issue cannot be followed blindly. You might 100% satisfy a program's criteria but yet you might not get the interview call. To get over this problem, information/advice from residents already in the system is very useful. There are certain good programs which regularly accept IMGS and there are others which don't, in spite of proclaiming that they accept FMGS and also sponsor Visas. Always ask seniors and residents, advice after you have shortlisted. Many programs ask for compulsory US Clinical Experience and yet call candidates without it for interviews. Another method is to check their website if they have FMGS in their program. However there are not many programs which have a list of their residents on their website. If email id is displayed of the FMG resident, then mail them and get the 'inside info'.

V. BY SEPTEMBER 1ST OF YEAR PRECEDING MATCH

Filling the Application Form: Filling the online application in myeras is quite simple. The following are some of the clarifications you will need.
a. Account–Profile: This is the only part of the application that you can update/ change later after submitting. Those of you who need a Visa to undergo residency training will need a H-1B or J1 Visa.
b. Application–CAF: Many questions pertaining to licensure, certification and membership apply to the US organizations and usually the answer will be 'NONE' for an IMG.
American Medical Graduates (AMG) after schooling need to undergo 4 years of Undergraduate studies before they enter medical school for another 4 years, so the answer to the column 'Education' will be 'None' for an IMG. Our CRRI/Internship in Medical School qualities as work experience.
c. Documents–LOR: You need to first designate the letter writer in the application. The LORS that you will mail to ECFMG will be uploaded to match with the designated Professor.
Personal Statement: Try to restrict yourself to 1 page in a word document using Font Size 12 in Times New Roman. Points that need to be addressed are :
  a. Why did you decide on a Medical Career?
  b. Why did you choose that particular Specialty?
  c. Why did you choose that particular Program?
  d. Details about your Medical Education.
Try to make it interesting and avoid too many 'I's.
USMLE Transcript: Eras will transmit your USMLE scores directly the first time you apply. You need to make a choice between automatic transmission and manually selecting the retransmit button for the future. In the former, once your exam result (e.g. Step 3) has been declared they will automatically transmit it to the programs you have applied to. In the latter case, you need to click on the retransmit button. The advantage of this is that you can choose not to transmit your result if you fail the exam (God forbid). However once you retake the exam and click on the retransmit button, both your present (pass) status and your previous failed report will be transmitted.
d. *Programs:* Search the programs and save the ones you are interested in. The Programs then move to the 'Selected' category. Go to the 'Apply to' category and apply to the selected programs. Before applying, your application should be 'Submitted'. Be careful before submitting as you cannot make any changes later. After submitting your application, apply to 1 program on September 1st. You will have to pay at this time.

The Nuts and Bolts of Residency Application 131

$ 60 – Eras Processing Fee
$ 50 – USMLE Transcript Fee.

Check in a day or 2 on ADTS (Applicant document and tracking system) (available as a link in the eras website) if your application is in the Postoffice. You can then apply to the rest of the programs. The $ 60 Eras Processing fee will cover your first 10 programs. The next 10 costs $ 8 each and the next 10, $ 15 each. After 30 programs every program will decrease the weight of your purse by $ 25. You can check on ADTS frequently if the programs are downloading your application. The Dean's letter however will be downloaded only in November/December.

Therefore the total expenditure for your application will be:

$ 75 – Eras Token fee
$ 60 – Eras Processing Fee
$ 50 – USMLE Transcript Fee
$ 65 – NRMP Registration Fee
+ The cost of applying to programs numbering greater than 10.

August 20th Post the Documents to ECFMG which need to be scanned and uploaded on to your online application. These include:

a. College Transcript
b. Dean's Letter/ MSPE
c. Letters of Recommendation
d. Colour photograph

One week to 10 days before you actually want to apply, post the documents, because it takes that long to scan and upload. After September 1st it takes progressively longer time to upload your documents. You can make sure if your documents have been uploaded by using ADTS. You can only see if the documents are uploaded but not the actual scanned documents.

About the letters of recommendation, a minimum of 4 are required. The number of recommendation letters required by each program varies from 2-4, the most common being 3. You can upload as many LOR as you want but can assign only a maximum of 4 to each program. Get your LOR early, as early as January of the previous year to the match. The following is an indication format for a LOR.

Name and: Home Address:
Designation: Home Phone:
Address of Medical: Cell Phone:
College/Hospital:
                                   E-mail ID:
Contact Number in the Hospital:

(Letter Head)

Points to be covered: (Body of Letter)
Communication skills
Bedside manners
Ability to work in a team
Pleasant personality
Extracurricular activities and of course about your academic record.

SIGNATURE
NAME AND DESIGNATION

Try to get LORS from Heads of Departments, Professors and Registrars. **Waiver** information on these Documents and where to post it to is available at the ECFMG Website under ERAS.

VI. SEPTEMBER 1 OF YEAR PRECEDING MATCH

Apply

Do not procrastinate. If you want a head start over others you need to do this. No point regretting later. Even a delay of 15 days makes a difference. Even after applying, you can upload more LORS, retransmit a new USMLE Score result, and change your 'MY PROFILE'.

How Many Programs to Apply to

A difficult and dicey question to answer. It depends on:
a. Your level of confidence if you can judge yourself well
b. Competitiveness that year
c. The field of your interest. For example. Psychiatry is easier to come by than Pediatrics than Internal medicine.
d. Your communication skills: This is important for the interviews. If you feel that your CS are not too good you could apply to more institutions just to increase the number of interviews and therefore your chances.
e. If you are applying to very competitive programs, obviously you need to increase their number to increase your chances. An average number is 40.

VII. USMLE STEP 3 EXAM

Step 3 Exam

Take it in, September, October. However it will be excellent if you are able to clear it before you apply. This will give you an edge over others with visa issues; H-1B Visa but not J1 visa.

Meanwhile by October 1st week start calling the programs you had applied to and ask for your application status. Some program coordinators can be rude but you have to take it in your stride. Try some excuse for calling them up for example, if you are recently ECFMG certified or have cleared your Step 3, to inform them and at the same time remind them of your application to their program.

VIII. NRMP REGISTRATION

PAY YOUR NRMP FEES; By December 1st @ the NRMP (National resident matching program) website, otherwise you will have to pay a penalty. Click on register and then applicant registration.

IX. THE INTERVIEW SEASON: NOV/DEC/(JAN) OF YEAR PRECEDING THE MATCH

A. Selection Criteria for interviews for an FMG

a. Any Visa issue — US citizens preferred over GC holders over H1/J1 candidates
b. US Clinical Exp — Has gained a lot of importance since last match
c. USMLE scores and your CV (publications, research, work experience)
d. Complete application form

B. What to do when you receive the interview call?

1. Send a thanks letter to the program coordinator or director.
2. Before calling them to set the date for interview, try to find out with the current residents or other people in the program about the psychology of the director in terms of earlier interview candidates and later candidates. Some programs have a tendency to select from earlier candidates and some have the opposite.
3. Before going to the interview, you should always try to find out about your specific interview board personnel and try to know their psychology. You should also know about their position in the program, their research interests

and if they have any recent publications. Sometimes they feel good if you have the same research interest as them and they start talking about it.
4. You should try to arrive at that city or the hospitals 2-3 days before the interview and speak with the chief resident, other residents and interns. When you are asked in the interview about the program, then always quote that you have been here for 2-3 days, observing the atmosphere with residents and you really like the place. Try to make friends with the Chief resident because one of the chief resident is also on the interview board.

PREPARE—research program, research interviewers, mock interviews, rehearse answers to common questions.

5. Arrange for accomodation and travel as detailed below

C. Scheduling the interviews

Schedule the interview at your convenience. Although the general idea is to schedule the good ones in January so that they remember you. My opinion is if they are impressed by you, they will remember you no matter what. Try to group the interviews areawise so that you don't have to travel unnecessarily. This is difficult but if you are expecting more interviews from that region then leave dates free around the one you have scheduled in that area. Schedule the good programs in which you are not very interested early so that you will get a feel of the interview process before you go on to ace them.

Very important: Schedule your interviews together.... download professional calender logs from the internet (which is what I did for free), download maps of the US from websites, maps that show all the cities and towns of all states (called the clickable or zoomable maps).

Start adding interview dates as they come.... name each week as the week of a state... for example, NY, Texas, Michigan, Illinois are like states where most IMGs will have interviews... plan to spend a full week in each state and schedule accordingly... Travel from state to state on weekends....depending on where you live.... Fly between the east coast to the midwest or the west coast and travel by other means from airport to the city/ town of interview...

The above explanation on scheduling is important because intelligent scheduling saves hundreds of dollars more than the "smart deals" of southwest...

D. How to travel to the interview?

1. AEROPLANES: If you have only a few interviews, scattered all over, (like 5-8 interviews), fly, with good deals and brought early, you can finish the travelling within $ 1000..... If you have lots of interviews, concentrated in

The Nuts and Bolts of Residency Application 135

one or two states, fly to one state and travel by other means to the city / town of interview. Lots of interviews, lots of money, fly....!

1. AIR TRAVEL MOST IMPORTANT: SEARCH WIDE, BOOK EARLY:
   southwest.com
   expedia.com
   travelocity.com
   bestprice.com
2. BUSES:
   greyhound.com

   Advantages:
   - very cheap
   - goes to every small town in the US
   - air conditioned
   - bathroom inside bus
   - Disadvantages:
   - long journeys
   - long layovers enroute
   - bathrooms stink
   - safe????

   TIP:
   - online reservation cheaper than tickets at station
3. THE BEST WAY TO TRAVEL
   TRAIN......... (Probably the best way to travel)
   amtrak.com

This travel is unlimited for a particular period of time in that geographic zone and the prices are lesses during off-peak periods.

E. How to prepare for the interview

This is the easiest of the entire ordeal, in contrast to how you feel before your first interview experience. So relax. First prepare answers to the common questions. Then get ready the things your need for the interview. Buy a suit (much cheaper in India) preferably dark colored and it could be a skirt for ladies. Wear formal shoes and carry a folder with all your documents. Present yourself neatly and professionally. You are not appearing for an exam as a student rather it's a job interview. Appear confident and articulate (I know that's tough !) with as many people as possible. Be congenial, pleasant and at the same time ask questions about the program. Remember the interviews are two way assessments. So ask questions, form an opinion and on getting back home jot down the pros and cons of the program as they will fade away quickly with subsequent interviews.

Subtleties of interviews...

1. Body language is very important.
2. Experienced interviewers put both chairs on the same side of the table.
3. Inexperienced ones sit on one side of a big table and let you sit on the other side.
4. Good programs try to impress you to rank them highly.
5. The bad programs ask medical questions and put the onus on you to impress them.
6. Use a standardized form to evaluate each program rather than go by gut feeling. (MUST/ WANT by Iserson's).
7. English and communication skills are very important.
8. Program coordinators rate you too… the first few minutes when you say hi and talk to them, you will see that they are evaluating you too. At UIC-Christ the PC fills out the form on you too.
9. The rank order list of the program is decided 50 % by your CV, etc and 50 % by your interview performance (I saw the form used at Christ, it asked the interviewer about scores, about English, communication skills, LORs, etc).
10. Closing part of the interview is very important.
11. If you are poor at interviewing, kindly have some mock interviews.

The programs judge you by spending a few hours with you. Put yourself in their shoes. Who will you be most impressed by. A communicative, friendly, pleasant person who gets along with most people. That is what you should aim for. It is your personality that they are looking at since your CV already reflects your academic achievements.

Research the program before you land for the interview. It makes a good impression. Pre-interview dinner is a casual occasion. Wear trousers and a sweater or a shirt. No need to carry your documents. You will meet the chief resident and other residents. You can ask questions about vacation time and no. of days off/week which you should not ask the Program Director. Also ask them about the working atmosphere, how much free time they get and do they get time to study. In the midst of this interaction eat well. Do not peck at your food; it might indicate that you are tensed. Most important–Be ontime. Use a checklist to create a uniform set of criteria for all the programs that you will be considering. This will help you to remember the details of each program and help you to formulate a complete picture of what is available.

Key point to get residency is that you have to be confident not arrogant, you have to be strong and enthusiastic not weak and indifferent, you have to give them an impression that you will get the residency anyway and you are here for just to evaluate the program. Don't feel weak and miserable be energetic and think positive. When your interview finishes the program should have an impression that you are a very strong candidate and if they miss you, they will make a big mistake.

Personal approach: meet people over there and try to show your face to the program director before the interview. Meet the chief resident and other residents. And ask the first year interns about the question of interview because they have gone through the same process.

Remember to always be neat and well groomed, but comfortable, when going for your interviews, Conservative dresses are still your best bet, so that means dark blazers, suits and dresses are appropriate. If interviewing on the east coast remember to dress warmly. Always arrive at your destination early.

In most cases you will be on unfamiliar territory, so arriving early gives you the opportunity to find your way around the area and become comfortable with your surroundings, the World Wide Web (WWW) has become a terrific source of information, especially about universities and teaching hospitals. You can often find an up-to-date phone directory. Campus map, and information about the surrounding community on a university's web site. Be prepared to ask and answer questions.

Safe Number

With around 10-12 interviews you will most probably match. There have been instances where people with just one interview have matched and in contrast 25 interviews and remained unmatched.

Commonly asked questions in the interview

Answer all questions as truthfully as possible, only then will your genuineness come across. Take your time in answering the questions. Think and then reply. They will not hurry you. This way you will not sound rehearsed and you will also have time to refine your answer. If you are asked an 'out of the blue' question do not panic, just think about it and you will salvage yourself.

a. Tell me about yourself—An open ended question for you to open up and also solves the interviewers problem of where and how to begin. This can be

answered in anyway you like. Give a brief summary of your education and your personality.
b. Why did you choose IM/Peds/Psychiatry….?
c. Why did you choose this particular program?
   I found this question the most difficult and it is frequently asked. They are very responsive if you know a resident in their program and thus applied. If not so, then praise the program, that you heard about it from your seniors and that it is a very good program.
d. Why did you choose to come to the US?
e. Difference in health care delivery between the US and your home country.
f. Your hobbies and interests.
g. Tell me about your graduate medical education.
h. Tell me about the last/any interesting case you have seen.
i. Are you interested in any particular fellowship?
   This is to find out if they can help you further in that specialty. Some programs even arrange the interviewer from that specialty. If you have not decided as yet, then frankly admit it.
j. Questions about your family, where you are staying in the US and your means of transport are common topics of getting to know you.
k. Why is there a gap between your graduate medical education and the present?
l. Be thorough with your CV as questions can be posed from any part.
m. What are your strengths and weaknesses?
n. What questions do you have?
o. Where else have you got interview calls from?

F. Questions that you can ask

Research the program before you land for the interview. It makes a good impression. Information is accessed from their website.
a. What are the rotations as an intern and as a resident? (An intern is a first year resident).
b. How frequent are the overnight calls for an intern?
c. How many days off/week and vacation time? (Ask the residents).
d. Do they follow the cap system?
   (Cap is the upper limit of the no. of patients up to which an intern/resident can take on).
e. How does the system work in the ICU—are there overnight calls?
f. Do they have the night float system?

Night Float—Many programs have one month of night duty and in such programs the residents do not do overnight calls but do short call up to 8 or 10 pm till the night float team takes over.
g. Do they allow 'moon lighting'?
Moonlighting is a means of earning extra money for the resident. Here the hospital asks for help from residents who are free (evenings or off period, etc.) when there is shortage of hands and pays them for it. Residents on J1 visa are not allowed to moonlight and certain programs do not allow even those on H1 to moonlight.
h. What is your patient population like?
i. How do they assess their residents?
j. What is the Day schedule like?
e.g. Morning Report - 7-8 am
Wards – 8-12
Noon Conference– 12-1
And so on.
k. Is the hospital completely computerized or should patient charts be filled by hand?
l. How are the library facilities?
m. No. of electives in the PGY1, 2, 3.
This is vital, cause if you are interested in a fellowship you need to apply for it at the end of the first year or by the middle of the II Year.
n. Is the atmosphere congenial in the hospital?
How is the resident—consultant relationship? How are the staff-nurses?
o. What is the housing like near the hospital? Is the area safe? How about public transport in the region?
p. How is the research activity in your program?
q. How many residents get into fellowships and where?
r. Does the program propagate attending conferences and do they fund for the same?

These questions start getting on your nerves after a few interviews. More so, cause you already know a lot about the program from researching. With time you will find it difficult to concentrate on and listen to the answers. But show that you are interested in and try to keep the conversation lively.

G. Few or no Interview What to do?

1. Ask myself: "WHY DIDN'T I GET ANY / MANY INTERVIEWS?"
There are many reasons for not getting interviews....

Do I have low scores? (below 80 or 85)
Do I have multiple attempts?
Do I have the ECFMG certificate?
Am I an old Grad (more than 5 years since graduation)
Have I taken my Step 3?
Do I have any USCE?
Do I have volunteer experiences?
Do I need a visa?
If yes, what kind of visa?
Do I have any research experience?
Do I have any LORs from US physicians?
Is my application suited to the specialty I am applying for?
Did I utilise my contacts to get observerships or externships?
Are there relatives/ friends or contacts who can get me interviews?
Are there errors or gaps in my transcript?
Is it possible for me to get an AAMC formatted Dean's letter or MSPE?
Do I have my medical school awards or honors?
Is my personal statement well written.... number of words, length, grammar, content, message?
Did I apply to a large number of programs (very important)?
Did I research programs before I applied?
Did I apply early enough to get interviews from community hospitals?
2. If you have no interviews or only close to five interviews, there is HIGH probability of going unmatched. Am I mentally prepared to face this possibility?
3. Do I stand a chance in the post match scramble.... if yes, what is the process, how am I going to do it... what documents do I need?
4. If post match scramble doesn't work, how can I know about vacant PGY-1 slots that I can fill..... from March to October, many PGY-1 slots will be vacant due to many reasons... do I know the websites, contacts and residents to get this valuable information...
5. If match, post match and vacant PGY-1 slots don't work, what can I do???????
  Improve your application.... if not ECFMG certified—complete the process, if not taken Step 3-prepare hard and take it and get good score, if no USCE-get Observership/externship have I asked my relatives/friends for help in getting these positions... Can I change my visa status... can I get a job to change from B1/ B2 to J1/ H-1B.... A CRA job or research job that sponsors a visa.... Doing research....related to your specialty....getting presentations or publications can take you places... and remember to emphasize them in your application and

The Nuts and Bolts of Residency Application   141

PS... Send thank you letter after the interview to the PD, all interviews and if possible go for a revisit. Might show has interested you are in the program.

The year of the match

X. PRE-MATCH OFFER

You might get this offer anytime between November and January. Pre-match offer is an out of match settlement. Match is a computerized process where the programs and the candidates submit their rank list and they are matched. There is a degree of uncertainty in this process. Pre-match circumvents this problem and you can make a choice to accept one of the many pre-match offers you may receive.

Advantages

a. No insomnia regarding match. Absolutely sure that you are joining that particular program. No problem of remaining unmatched.
b. Helps in early processing of the visa so that you can join on time.

Disadvantages

a. May not be your Rank 1 program. If you refuse the pre-match, then may be, just may be, you have a chance with your better ranked ones.

The pre-match contract once signed is binding. Legal issues will result if you change your mind after signing the contract.

XI. RANK ORDER LIST DEADLINE

SUBMIT ROL (Rank Order List)

This is done in your account in NRMP. The last date is around February 3rd week. They will send you an email regarding the deadline. You can start ranking from January middle.

How to rank

Do not care about what the programs think of you or your status in their rank order list (ROL). Rank them in order of your preference. If your Rank 1 program is top notch and you think that your performance at the interview was not up to your standard, still rank them number 1. This way you will still have a chance however small to match there versus forfeiting it by ranking it low or not at all.

More info in 'Match Algorithm' in NRMP website.

Do not rank a program you do not like, because the match is binding and if you break the bond you cannot participate in the match for the next few years.

The NRMP account is quite user-friendly. You can browse the programs (using the 'directory') participating in the match where details about how many positions are open are available. The nrmp/program number code for each program here is different from the number code in my eras when you apply which is the ACGME code. If you are unable to find a program in the site then it is not participating in the match. Do not forget to certify your ROL. You can change your ROL up to the deadline date but do not forget to click on the certify button every time.

XII. MATCH WEEK

This will fall in the middle of March. Prior to this NRMP, ERAS and AAMC will send you mails about how to rank and about post match scramble. If you receive the latter e-mail do not worry. There are rumors that if you receive that mail you will not match. This is a Rumour.

The time table of the Match Week will be up on the NRMP website.

MONDAY - 12 noon eastern time (New York Time) Candidates will know if
They have matched but not where they have matched.

TUESDAY - 12 noon Eastern Time–Scramble begins for those who did not match.
The list of unfilled positions is also available at this time. The Scramble goes on for 2 days.

THURSDAY - 1 pm eastern time – Match Day – Results of where you matched is Displayed.

Information on whether you matched and where is displayed in your NRMP account.

XIII. POST MATCH SCRAMBLE

This is a savior for those who did not match. Do not lose hope. Remaining unmatched is not a life-death problem. Take time to get back to normalcy and then start working on the scramble. Unmatched candidates will be issued the unmatched positions and those positions can be applied to. Once the scramble period (2 days) draws to a close, the remaining vacant positions can be retrieved from findaresident.com. You can continue to search for a position till June. Do not lose hope if it is not successful. There are still plenty more 'matches' and other hidden opportunities out there in the world.

Prepare to some extent for the scramble before the match irrespective of your confidence level. There are 4 ways of communicating to the programs with unfilled positions during the scramble period. They are:

a. E-mail
b. Myeras
c. Fax
d. Telephonic conversation

They are in descending order of difficulty. For emailing your details scan and ready your CV, personal statement, USMLE score report and a covering letter stating your interest in the program and your USMLE scores and if ECFMG certified.

You can apply through my ERAS up to a maximum of 30 programs. You cannot reapply to a program during the scramble if you had already applied to it during the matching season. In such cases you should call them or email them to let them know that they already have your application through ERAS.

Telephonic conversation is the best but it will be difficult to contact the program as the lines will be busy. The best procedure is to call the programs, letting them know that you are interested in and asking them as to how to send in your application. You can fax it once they say so. If lines are busy start emailing and apply through my ERAS. Addresses and contact information are available at 'Frieda'.

SUMMARY

As discussed in the introduction, from June of the year before the match, you must have your USMLE Step 1 and 2 CK scores, take Step 2 CS in July so tat you get your result in September, do research/ Observership or USCE before August, get presentations, publications or letters of recommendation that can strengthen your application, get your ERAS token in July, fill out the MYERAS application form and, send your documents to ECFMG by August, research and choose list of programs you want to apply and have everything ready by September 1st. On September 1st, apply. Wait for interview calls and have a back up plan if you do not have many interviews. Prepare and plan for interview and interviews at different programs. Register with NRMP by December 1st and rank programs based on your preference by Feb 23rd. Await your match results on March 16th.

Web sites

www.residencyandfellowship.com
www.aippg.com.info/residencyinterview.html
www.medstudent.ucla.edu
www.sentwork.com

REFERENCES

http://www.aamc.org/audienceeras.htm
http://www.nrmp.org
http://www.amtrak.com
http://www.greyhound.com

Section Six
Customizing Your Application for Your Specialty

Internal Medicine

Vijayprasad Gopichandran, Nirav Mamdani

INTRODUCTION

"The eye does not see what the mind does not know"—Sir William Osler.

This statement could not be more suitable for any field other than Internal Medicine, with its myriad fantasies and abstract presentations. Each day for the internist is a new day and each patient is a new challenge. This broad and all encompassing field of medicine catering from the adolescent to the elderly is very important and significant. For international medical graduates who enter the United States for training, this is the most popular field of choice. Internal Medicine is like the mother bird with wide wings, taking all the younglings under her feathers and nurturing them into specialists and super specialists. This chapter is an overview of Internal Medicine as a choice of specialization, its characteristic features, the international medical graduates scenario, the process of applying and getting into residency, the life during internal medicine residency and career options after the training in Internal Medicine.

Internal Medicine by Choice or by Chance

Making a decision to do Internal Medicine residency is a matter of personal choice. The attributes of Internal Medicine as a specialty, which attracts doctors to choose it, are:
1. Intellectually challenging.
2. Involving deductive reasoning.
3. Abstract conceptualization.
4. Broad-based, encompassing many organ systems and specialties.

148 Acing the USMLE and the Match

5. Providing wide options for specialization.
6. Physically and emotionally less demanding than specialties like trauma, emergency, surgery, etc.
7. Scope for academic pursuits.

But not many of us get the opportunity to make this choice. For many of us Internal Medicine happens more due to chance than due to choice. The high feasibility factor of obtaining an Internal Medicine residency as an international medical graduate makes many of us land up in internal medicine without a conscious choice. The next few paragraphs will outline the features of Internal Medicine residency and make this decision (whether by choice or by chance) a more meaningful one.

COMPETITIVENESS OF SPECIALTY

Internal Medicine—The IMG Scenario

Let us take a look at some important points about Internal Medicine residency training in the United States. Table 17.1 gives some statistics about Internal Medicine residency from the year 2004.

Table 17.1: Internal medicine residency statistics

1. Number of accredited Internal Medicine Program in the US: 387
2. Length of accredited training: 3 years
3. Average Number of Interviews conducted per program per year: 195.3
4. Total Number of active residents and fellows in training: 21,332

Since Internal Medicine is the launch pad for training into several specialties, which are associated with it, it is the most popular residency program. It has the highest number of active residents and interns in training at any point. Table 17.2 demonstrates the striking difference in the numbers of active residents and fellows in training in various specialties.

Table 17.2: Active residents and fellows in training in various specialties

S. No	Specialty	Number of active residents and fellows in training in the year 2004
1.	Internal Medicine	21,332
2.	Family Practice	9,373
3.	Pediatrics	7,811
4.	General Surgery	7,689
5.	Obstetrics and Gynecology	4,703
6.	Psychiatry	4,563

Contd...

Contd...

S. No	Specialty	Number of active residents and fellows in training in the year 2004
7.	Radiology	4,160
8.	Emergency Medicine	4,096
9.	Pathology	2,255
10.	Neurology	1,368
11.	Ophthalmology	1,274
12.	Otolaryngology	1,090

Given the large numbers of potential spots to be filled in by residents and fellows, Internal Medicine offers the fertile ground for most of the international medical graduates. It would not be far away from the truth to say, "All IMGs are in internal medicine unless proved otherwise"!!! There are about 11,000 international medical graduates in training in Internal Medicine and its related specialties each year.

International Medical Graduates in the US pursue their training on either a J1 Visa or an H-1B Visa. Some of them possess permanent resident status and some of them are citizens. It is essential to know which program supports which type of Visa and apply to the appropriate programs. Usually J1 and H-1B are the most common visa types. H-1B is the most preferred due to the ease of immigration possibilities. The pros and cons of these visas are discussed elsewhere in the book. The list of programs sponsoring J1 and H-1B Visas are available in several forms. It would also be advisable to check with the individual programs before applying to them.

APPLYING TO PROGRAMS—INDIVIDUALISING CURRICULUM VITAE AND PERSONAL STATEMENT

The Application Process: Curriculum Vitae

As described elsewhere in the book, the vital aspect of the application for any residency is the curriculum vitae. This is no exception for the Internal Medicine application. Specific guidelines to preparing a good curriculum vitae may be sought in other chapters in this book. At this point it may suffice to say that the following features are the highlights of a curriculum vitae for an internal medicine applicant:
1. Demonstration of a commitment to academics:
   - Research
   - Publications

- Presentations
- Teaching
- Participation in learning activities like CME
2. Good Scores in USMLE and academic track record.
3. Well-rounded personality.
4. Wide and varied interests.
5. Specific focused activities in internal medicine related fields if available.

For example, a CV containing evidence of active participation in clinical meetings and journal clubs would demonstrate commitment to academic pursuits and make the application stronger. Focused research in cardiology would not only strengthen the application for internal medicine residency but it also adds value for future fellowship opportunities. If one plans to apply for more than one specialty it is better to have more than one curriculum vitae tailor made for each of the programs. But unfortunately the ERAS does not allow this. Therefore it would be prudent to appropriately highlight the features that are important for the specialty that one prefers the most.

The Application Process—Personal Statement

It would not be an exaggeration if it is said that the single most important document which decides the fate of a wannabe internal medicine resident in the US is the personal statement. An ideal internal medicine personal statement contains details such as:

1. Why do I want to do internal medicine?
2. What are my attributes which make me suitable for internal medicine?
3. What are the opportunities that I have had which have molded my interest in internal medicine?
4. What do I plan in the future after internal medicine?
5. Why do I prefer to do it in this particular program? (Preferable to have individually tailored statements for each program applied, if possible!)

The internal medicine personal statement should highlight the features and characteristics that one possesses which cannot be described in the curriculum vitae. For example, one might be extremely good at communication skills; this can be described in the form of anecdotes and examples in the personal statement. This would add weight to the application. Needless to say that the combination of a good curriculum vitae and a good personal statement is a must for obtaining an interview with a residency program.

INTERVIEWING IN YOUR SPECIALTY

The Internal Medicine Residency Interview

The general features of typical residency interviews, the interview taking tips and other details are described elsewhere in the book. This chapter will focus on the Internal Medicine interview. The internal medicine interview differs from others in that there is a greater possibility of subject-based questions to be asked than during a typical surgical or obstetric interview. Given the broad base of the specialty the interviewer might be either a cardiologist, a nephrologists, a rheumatologist or some other specialist with his/her own inherent biases and prejudices. The cornerstone of the interview as in any other is making the first impression that the applicant is suitable for the considered program. Confidence and honesty as always are the benchmarks of a good interview.

RANK ORDER LIST

This is very straightforward. Rank as per your preference. Do not get influenced by the rumor that inevitably floats around every year advising candidates to rank programs based on the probability of the program picking you. Rank every program that you interview at even if you have too many interviews.

DURING RESIDENCY IN YOUR SPECIALTY

Life during Internal Medicine Residency

It is often quoted and almost always complained that an intern has no 'life'. This is true for a large part but the scenario is rapidly changing with the 80 hours work week rules in the US. Among the specialties the relatively easier and physically and emotionally less demanding one is internal medicine. According to a statistical report the average hours of work per week for a typical internal medicine resident is 64.8 and the average maximum consecutive hours on duty is 27.4. As an internal medicine resident one on an average gets one day of the week off. These statistics are relatively tighter in more competitive and busier programs. The average resident/fellow's salary during the residency is about $ 40,000 per annum.

Books for Internal Medicine Residency

Here is my perspective

- Uptodate is the main source of recent evidence-based information, and also quick reference when you are unsure of something during patient care. It is

also a good start point if you want to do some review type of research on some topic. Eventually you will have to go to pubmed for research, but using uptodate as a start point always helped me.
- Washington Manual (some people use Ferri's, but I thought it was more for med students and Wash manual is for residents/interns) is a very useful thing to have in your pocket, particularly when on call. It has detailed info as to exactly what to do in management of various problems. If you have ready access to uptodate, you may not need Wash manual too often, but still good idea to have it.
- Reading journals (New England Journal of Medicine being my journal of choice), review articles, journal clubs and other evidence-based sources would train you how to interpret various research articles/evidence-based information and use it in clinical practice. Many programs (including mine) have their own evidence-based medicine learning courses.
- MKSAP and MedStudy are the corner stones of board exams. Remember preparation of board exam does not start in third year!! It starts from the first day of your internship, and I will highly recommend reading these sources right from beginning.
- Keep one textbook as reference: some people like Harrison's, some CMDT and others Cecil. You will not be able to read more than one textbook and also it is not required. So stick to one text, preferably one that you used in your medschool.
- Much of the learning in residency comes through practical experience, morning reports, rounds and grand rounds. For me, practical experience and morning reports were the two most important sources of learning and will highly recommend to everyone to attend as many morning reports as you can. Case-based learning is the gist of residency.

All in all: Do not stress out about reading during residency, you will surely learn a lot during residency, but reading would be just one of the ways knowledge comes. (until now, books were the main, if not only, source). There is no need to read anything now, just relax till your residency starts!! Enjoy as much as you can!

Remember it is completely my own personal opinion based on my own experience till the end of third year of residency, and each and every one of you will actually develop your own way of acquiring knowledge.

SPECIALISATION AFTER RESIDENCY

After the Internal Medicine Residency

About 7000 internal medicine residents graduate from the residency each year. There are several possible tracks these graduates take for a career. About 50% of

Internal Medicine

them go for fellowship training. About 30% take to practice and the remaining take to careers as academicians. The most popular option is pursuing of fellowship training. The flowchart given in Figure 17.1 reproduced from "Creating a New National Workforce for Internal Medicine"—a position paper of the American College of Physicians, 2006 written by M Reene Zerehi, depicts the various career choices available for the graduates of an internal medicine residency program.

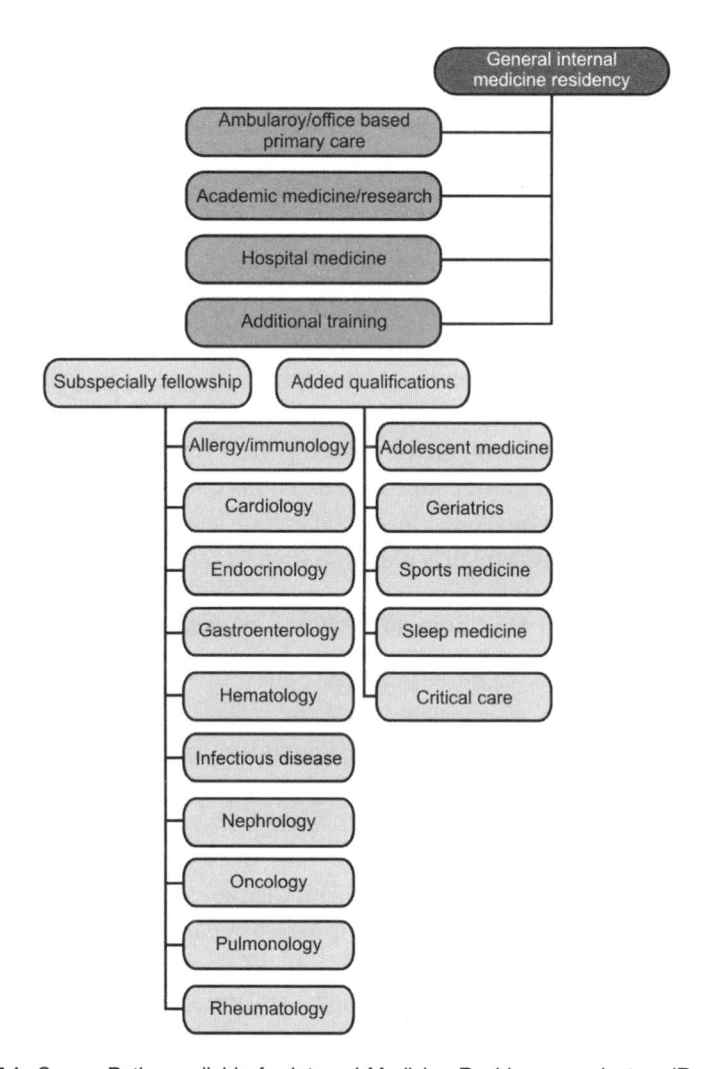

Figure 17.1: Career Paths available for Internal Medicine Residency graduates. (Reproduced from "Creating a New National Workforce for Internal Medicine. American College of Physicians, A Position Paper 2006 by M Renee Zerehi.)

WHAT AFTER IM RESIDENCY?

There are two options:

1. Do the residency, get the green card and then go for fellowship. Easiest from the standpoint of immigration issues, but once you have a gap, it becomes difficult to get into fellowship. You lose contacts and "stream of training". Overall, it looks a better option but it is not, at least I believe that. I have seen so many people deciding that and then not getting into fellowship for one reason or the other. It is also difficult to redirect your lifestyle back to fellowship.
2. Second option is to go for fellowship right after the residency on H1 visa and then to go for green card. It is easy to get fellowship right after as you are in contact with many people and they know you. Programs also prefer to take people right after residency. The negatives of this approach are two: you will need a program for fellowship that sponsors H1 visa and second problem is at the end of fellowship. Most competitive fellowships are for three years and that way you use all six years of H1 visa. That means, you will have to find a sponsor right after you fellowship for green card, and that should preferably be filed before the end of your fifth year of fellowship, which is difficult to do. If you don't find sponsor right after, the other option is to go back to your home country (or any other country, does not have to be your home country, just outside the US) for one year and that resets H1 clock for another six years which is plenty of time to get green card.

Summary of Internal Medicine as a choice of residency training

1. Internal medicine is the easiest residency program to get into as an international medical graduate.
2. It is a broad-based and general specialty and has good scope for specialization in several fields.
3. Doctors who have an intellectual bent of mind, interest for abstract reasoning, less preference for active and "on the toes" work environment and widely varied interests best suit into internal medicine.
4. But many times internal medicine happens by chance rather than choice for international medical graduates.
5. The life of an internal medicine resident is relatively easier compared to the other specialties in terms of physical and emotional stress.
6. Opportunities for practice and for further training are galore.

Salary Profile

The average annual salary for an internist without specialization is $ 1,62,000.

REFERENCES

http://www.ama-assn.org/vapp/freida/spcstsc/0,1238,140,00.html—Internal Medicine Specialty Training Statistics.

http://www.acponline.org/college/pressroom/as06/workforce_paper.pdf — "Creating a New National Workforce for Internal Medicine. American College of Physicians, A Position Paper 2006 by M Renee Zerehi.

http://www.ama-assn.org/vapp/freida/career/0,1238,140,00.html—Internal Medicine Graduates' Career Plan Statistics.

Pediatrics

Chandrasekhar Yangalsetty

INTRODUCTION

Pediatrics is an established IMG-friendly specialty in the US. While most Pediatric residency programs select their candidates *via* ERAS and NRMP, it is a fact that some reputed programs select their candidates out of match (non-competitive/pre-match). This is good news, for IMG candidates with experience. They will be offered pre-match if Institution thinks they are too precious to lose in Match. Pediatrics is not the best paid specialty as it is in developing countries like India. However, currently there is great demand for Pediatricians in the USA and this is expected to last at least a decade. It is probably easiest specialty to obtain a job, and also for J1 visa holders it is one of the easiest specialties to get a Waiver job. Pediatrics is mostly preventive pediatrics in the USA, with stress on developing strategies to prevent illness.

COMPETITIVENESS OF SPECIALTY

Pediatrics is a relatively non-competitive specialty in the United States.

APPLYING TO PROGRAMS—INDIVIDUALISING CURRICULUM VITAE AND PERSONAL STATEMENT

Applying to programs

Which programs to apply depends on one's scores, and the experience. A person with MD in Pediatric medicine, and Institutional experience should be on the lookout for a University program which has few sub-specialty fellowships. It is easier to get into fellowships in the same university than a university of another place or any other institution in a different place. A person with lower scores and reasonable experience (not qualified) should opt for City hospitals. A person with high scores but no/negligible experience should opt both for University programs and also for the City hospitals as they stand a chance of getting selected in either of the places. Qualification like a Residency in Pediatrics increases the individual's preferences. Programs can be choosen depending on their location and reputation. Another important thing to look for in a Pediatrics program is the subspecialty representation it has, in terms of the faculty and rotations available. For example, someone interested in pursuing a fellowship in Neonatology should find out more about the experience in NICU residency program offers. Among subspecialties for Pediatrics, Cardiology and Genetics are most difficult to get into and also highest paid. Neonatology and Infectious diseases, pulmonology are relatively easier to get into and are reasonably well paid. Most fellowships, if not all do not sponsor H-1B visas for the candidates. That leaves one with the option of taking a J1 visa at the outset that is while starting the residency. The only other way of getting into fellowship after finishing residency is possessing either EAD or green card. Obviously, if one is a citizen, then also programs accept you into fellowships. Contrary to the popular belief, J1 Visa is the safest method to finish the residency and to get into fellowship. Also eventually every IMG will end up with the green card as the USA is very reluctant to lose a US trained doctor. So it all boils down to one thing. What do you want? A green card 2 years earlier and not doing fellowship or getting into fellowship and getting green card a couple of years later. Also this affects in the family economics in the sense as J2 candidate gets work permit and is allowed to work. If you are on H-1B, as your spouse he/she will be H4 and will not be allowed to work. According to my experience as an IMG, one should apply at least 40 to 60 programs to expect some interview calls. Don't be afraid to sell yourself and keep applying to the highly reputed programs irrespective of your scores, especially if you have good institutional experience of considerable duration.

INTERVIEWING IN YOUR SPECIALTY

The interview

After applying to your desired programs, wait for the interview invitations which may come via regular mail, email or rarely via telephone. Contrary to the popular belief, don't wait too long to schedule your interview with the hospital. My suggestion is to get the earliest date possible. Of course you should be ready. There is no way you can improve your performance in a week's time as it is intended to look at your personality and they will exactly do that. Mind you they are experienced in doing that and they could hardly be fooled. Be yourself is the best advice I can give you. In trying to be unnatural, you can make a fool of yourself and lose a position which was definitely in reach. Most interviewers make you feel comfortable, so not performing because of excessive tension does not arise. Get prepared for common questions like, Why do you like Pediatrics, and if you are changing your specialty, What makes you change your specialty at this juncture, Where do you see yourself five years from now, what prompts you to choose our Institute, that kind of stuff. It is better to rehears the answers well, at the same time sounding as natural as possible. The myth among Indian students is that, one has to be fluent and should speak very fast to impress these Caucasians, Completely untrue. On the contrary they will NOT be able to understand you, if you speak the way you speak in India. Give appropriate pauses, speak grammatically correct English, and look the interviewer in the eye. Don't ever make the mistake of arguing with the interviewer and tell your point of view and then shrug your shoulders. Thank before leaving and express your confidence of hearing from them at the earliest possible.

RANK ORDER LIST

This is very straightforward. Rank as per your preference. Do not get influenced by the rumor that inevitably floats around every year advising candidates to rank programs based on the probability of the program picking you. Rank every program that you interview at even if you have too many interviews.

SPECIALISATION AFTER RESIDENCY

Social pediatrics, aimed at reducing and preventing child abuse has a great deal of application. Behavioral pediatrics is the emerging specialty which has the goal of reducing conditions like ADHD, Autism, etc. One has to apply for the fellowships in the start of 2nd year and should secure a position to get into fellowship after the residency. Cardiology and Genetics are most competitive and well paid fellowships for Pediatrics. The available fellowships are:
- Cardiology
- Neurology
- Pulmonology
- Critical care medicine
- Infectious diseases
- Genetics
- Emergency medicine

- Adolescent medicine
- Developmental (behavioral) pediatrics
- Movement disorders
- Epilepsy
- Gastroenterology
- Hematology-oncology

SALARY PROFILES AND LIFESTYLE ISSUES

200,000 to 240,000 $ per annum is the initial salary for the sub-specialist. The median expected salary for a typical Pediatrician in the United States is $144,000.

[19] Psychiatry

Aditi Malik

INTRODUCTION

Psychiatry residencies in the US have always been IMG friendly. The health care system is heavily dependent on IMG's as one third of all psychiatry slots are filled by us. A total of 983 graduates entered PGY1 general psychiatry residency programs in July 2006 out of which 340 were IMG's. The length of the program is usually 4 years but if you are interested in Child Psychiatry fellowship it can be done as 3 years of general psychiatry plus 2 years of fellowship. All other fellowships are a year long.

Psychiatry is a little different than other residencies as you really have to want to do it.

There are many challenges an IMG faces even after getting through the thick jungle of the USMLE's and the match. You are faced with the intersecting challenges of professional, personal and family acculturation. These challenges are significantly enhanced in psychiatry as you deal with cultural issues on an everyday basis. For example, your personal opinion on homosexuality or pedophilia will actually affect your professional life unlike if you were say, a surgical resident.

Future prospects in terms of **Clinical opportunities** include private practice in solo or group settings; working as an employee in a managed care or government setting; or becoming a supervisor or administrator. There is a tremendous need for **academic psychiatrists**, both clinician-educators and researchers. In the public arena, psychiatrists can become active in the community or government as advocates for mental health.

According to the American Psychiatric Association, there are approximately 39,000 psychiatrists and another 6,000 child psychiatrists for a total of 45,000, making psychiatry the fourth largest medical specialty.

COMPETITIVENESS OF SPECIALTY

Competitiveness for Psychiatry residency was Intermediate for the 2004 to 2006 match. Competitiveness is based on the percentage of US seniors who match in each specialty. Your CV and personal statement are of vital interest to the Residency Directors especially in psychiatry. After evaluating recommendations, transcripts, and test scores *ad nauseum*, busy Program Directors use the residency personal statement and CV to decide between applicants with very similar backgrounds and USMLE scores. A strong residency statement can help you land an interview; a weak one will ensure that you don't.

APPLYING TO PROGRAMS—INDIVIDUALISING CURRICULUM VITAE AND PERSONAL STATEMENT

Applying to Programs

There are several criteria to keep in mind when looking for a residency program. Obviously there are many factors to consider, many of which may be more important to you than these more readily quantifiable measures. A few factors that many consider important warrant discussion.

Lifestyle: Lifestyle factors include call-schedules and total number of work hours, salary in relation to local cost of living, moonlighting opportunities, and the cultural environment of the residency program and its community context. Call schedule and total number of work hours is of obvious interest to most would be residents. Psychiatry residency programs generally require fewer calls than most medical residencies.

Clinical training: Most residents planning a career in psychiatry value balanced clinical training emphasizing both psychopharmacology and psychotherapy. The emphasis by most programs these days is on a Biopsychosocial approach. However it's a good question to ask when selecting a program. If there is a chance you may want to pursue sub-specialty training, it will be important for you to consider availability of elective rotation exposure to fellowship-training in the sub-specialty you are interested in. Such exposure will be a valuable asset when you apply to fellowship training programs in the same sub-specialty. If you have no idea what sub-specialty you may be interested in, a program offering a wide variety of fellowship-training programs may be valuable to you.

Research opportunities: Responses from residency training directors and department heads to residency applicants striving for a research career are almost uniformly positive. Nevertheless, there are obvious differences in the research opportunities available across training programs. In general, programs that derive a large portion of their departmental budget from research funding are more likely to offer residents significant time away from clinical responsibilities to conduct their research. University programs such as University of Pittsburg, University of California San Diego, and Stanford University are often able to offer applicants the equivalent of approximately one full year of time dedicated to research during their four years of psychiatry residency training.

Work environment culture: You will be working with people involved with the residency you select for a minimum of four years. The individuals involved with each residency program help create a unique cultural environment, which in turn tends to help attract other people to the program who for various reasons are drawn to that particular kind of culture. For example, is the work environment culture warm and friendly or cool and distant? Is it "easygoing" or high pressured? In short, consider what kind of experience it will be to work with the people involved with residency training program including residents, faculty and administrative staff.

Institutional pedigree: Completing training at a big name university may provide some additional career flexibility at the beginning of your career, at least in academic psychiatry. Obviously, the work you do (i.e. in an academic career: the manuscripts you publish and the grant funding you obtain) will define your career and will quickly dwarf your training program pedigree in importance as you forge your career path. Be careful not to place too much importance in the name of institution where you wish to train at the expense of other factors you may, in the long run, find are more important when selecting the best residency training program "fit" for yourself.

Location: While it is true that the majority of physicians procure employment in or near the area where they completed their residency, this does not suggest it is impossible to find a good job elsewhere. Nevertheless, residents are likely to catch first wind of upcoming jobs near where they are training and may have already worked at the location where new jobs are being filled. Give the location due consideration.

Your residency statement must address why you became interested in psychiatry, what you can contribute to a given program, and how you intend to realize your professional goals. In addition, you must convincingly present evidence of your intellectual and personal credentials while demonstrating your motivation, determination, integrity, common sense, reliability, and personal capacity to excel in a challenging residency program. IMG candidates also must establish their English language ability.

My Personal statement is attached here for reference purposes.

Your CV should be crisp and to the point. Highlight important achievements and also your experiences in the field of psychiatry. A two page long CV is what you should aim for as people have short attention span. A few categories that you should cover in your CV are:

1. Demographic data
2. Education
3. Memberships in Honorary/Professional Societies
4. Research Experience
5. Volunteer Experience
6. Language Fluency
7. Computer Skills
8. Interests and Hobbies.

There were 181 psychiatry residency training programs accredited by the ACGME for 2005/2006. A list of these can be seen at this link http://www.ama-assn.org/vapp/freida/pgmrslt/1,1239,,00.html.

Some of the residency programs which were sponsoring H-1B visa for the 2005-2006 Match are as follows. This is not a complete list. So also do your own research. (This information is subject to change and should be verified with the program).

> University of Missouri at Kansas City
> St Luke's-Roosevelt Hospital Center
> Drexel U Coll of Med/MCP Hahnemann
> Case Western Reserve U (Metro Health)
> Mount Sinai School of Med (Elmhurst)
> Mount Sinai School of Medicine
> Albert Einstein Medical Center
> Brookdale University Hospital and Medical Ctr
> Albert Einstein COM—Montefiore Med Ctr
> Cleveland Clinic Foundation
> University of Missouri—Columbia Program
> SUNY Health Science Center at Brooklyn
> Albert Einstein Coll of Med—LI Jewish Med Ctr
> SUNY at Buffalo Graduate Medical—Dental
> St. Elizabeths Hospital, Washington DC

Other IMG friendly programs are listed below. These do sponsor only J1 visas
> Yale-New Haven Medical Center

Michigan State University
Northeastern Ohio Univ College of Med
John Peter Smith Hosp/Tarrant County Hosp
New York Medl College at Westchester Medical Ctr
West Virginia University (Charleston)
Albert Einstein COM at Bronx-Lebanon
University of South Dakota
U of Texas Health Sci Ctr (San Antonio)
West Virginia University
Penn State U/Milton S Hershey Med Ctr
University of Texas at Houston
University of North Dakota
Thomas Jefferson University
Kalamazoo Ctr for Med Studies/MSU
Jamaica Hospital Medical Center
Advocate Lutheran General Hospital Program
University of Texas Medical Branch Hospitals
Ohio State University Hospital Program
Eastern Virginia Medical School
Allegheny General Hospital Program
Finch Univ of Health Sciences/Chicago Med Sc
Bergen Regional Medical Center
Wayne State University/Detroit Medical Ctr
SUNY Upstate Medical University
St Louis University School of Medicine
University of Rochester
Loyola University
UMDNJ-Robert Wood Johnson Med School (Piscataway)
New York Med College (Richmond)
Indiana University School of Medicine
University of Connecticut
Institute of Living/Hartford Hospital
Virginia Commonwealth University Health System
Morehouse School of Medicine
Nassau University Medical Center

Some useful links and resources
Getting into a Residency, A Guide for Medical Students, by Kenneth V Iserson, MD, published by Galen Press, Ltd.

How to Choose A Medical Specialty, by Anita D Taylor, published by WB Saunders Company.

Resumes and Personal Statements For Health Professionals, by James W Tysinger, PhD, published by Galen Press, Ltd.

www.nrmp.org

http://www.psych.org/edu/careers.cfm

http://www.imgi.net

INTERVIEWING IN YOUR SPECIALTY

The interview

This is not to stereotype anyone but the ability to communicate with others and be comfortable in our own skin, are sometimes lacking in IMG's. Psychiatry programs are concerned with the person, not the board scores. Psychiatry revolves around the ability to communicate with people, and therefore that's what programs want. If you have exceptional scores in Step 1 but you cannot communicate effectively, most programs would be hesitant to rank you. Furthermore, if you failed Step 1 a few times and barely passed but are easy to talk to, make people feel at ease around you, programs will gobble you up. I have come to this conclusion after my own experience and from talking to friends in other programs that psychiatry selection is very unlike other fields.

Usually the interview is in a relaxed conversation form. I did not face any clinical questions during my interviews. Before you go for the interview, try thinking up replies to obvious questions you might be asked. For example—"Why did you decide to do psychiatry?" This saves you from stuttering and getting anxious on your big day. Review your CV and personal statement, know what's in there. There is nothing more embarrassing than looking clueless about something you wrote yourself. Get to know about the program that you are going to interview at so you can tailor your responses. If you know which faculty members will be interviewing you beforehand, Google them and try to learn what their interests are, as those can be springboards for interesting discussions. Do read a little bit about the history of psychiatry.

On the day of the interview dress conservative, tasteful, and comfortable. Organize the documents you would need. It's a good idea to write down the questions you would want to ask from the faculty and residents at the program. Another weak point for the IMG is that they are not used to asking questions of authority figures. However, do not ask questions related to salary, benefits, maternity leaves and vacations. These will be listed in the brochures that you will receive. Do not hesitate in asking for a tour of the area.

You may wish to thank the program coordinator before you leave for the well organized trip. It is a very good idea to send a thank you letter to everyone you interviewed with. It is going to be much easier if you write your thank you letter right after the interview while everything is fresh. Touch the subjects you talked about; that will make it more personal and your interest more genuine.

Why psychiatry interviews are tough…

1. The most important question in the interview is the question, "WHY PSYCHIATRY"… especially for IMGs who are interviewing in Psychiatry as a back up, it is essential to have a convincing answer. Even for someone like me with Psychiatry clinical experience, research trial in psychiatry and international presentation in Bulgaria with Best Paper award, it is a tough question to answer. So be prepared and speak convincing… if a psychiatric interviewer cannot pick up you are lying (especially a psychoanalytic psychiatrist or a forensic psychiatrist), no one can.
2. Another common question… and an important one at that is the question, "tell me about yourself"… it is very important to have a clear opinion about self and a good understanding about self… so the way this question is answered will largely decide whether you are ranked or not.
3. Another important question is, "what are your interests outside of Medicine"… again psychiatrists expect prospective psychiatrists to be well-rounded with active interests outside of Medicine.
4. In psychiatry, the faculty members do this all their life… interviewing is the BASIS and cornerstone of psychiatry… so when I come to recruitment of residents in psychiatry, they are natural… they know what to ask, how to evaluate and are less likely to be cheated.
5. A clear career focus is again more important in psychiatry than any other field… especially fellowship interests, areas of interest and research interests.
6. The interview plays a much important role in the rank order list than any other part of the process… for example, in Internal Medicine; the rank order list is decided 50 % by your ERAS application and 50% by your interview. In psychiatry, the rank order list would be in the range of 80% interview and 20% with the ERAS application.
7. Scores are not at all important in Psychiatry… they don't want 99/99/99 ERAS in Psychiatry, they need applicants who have an interest in Psychiatry or have demonstrated an interest in Psychiatry in the past.

RANK ORDER LIST

Preparing your rank order list

This is very straightforward. Rank as per your preference. Do not get influenced by the rumor that inevitably floats around every year advising candidates to rank programs based on the probability of the program picking you. Rank every program that you interview at even if you have too many interviews.

DURING RESIDENCY IN YOUR SPECIALTY

SPECIALISATION AFTER RESIDENCY

Some fellowships which can be done after Psychiatry Residency.

Subspecialty/fellowship training following completion of a psychiatry residency training program is available in addiction psychiatry, child and adolescent psychiatry, forensic psychiatry, geriatric psychiatry, pain management, and psychosomatic medicine. Detailed information about the scope of these subspecialty training programs, number of positions offered and length of training is available in the GMED (FREIDA).

Fellowships

Subspecialty	Length
Addiction Psychiatry	1 year
Child and Adolescent Psychiatry	2 years
Forensic Psychiatry	1 year
Geriatric Psychiatry	1 year
Pain Management	1 year
Psychosomatic Medicine	1 year

SALARY PROFILES AND LIFESTYLE ISSUES

The annual salary for psychiatrists ranges from $144,332 to $183,332. The median expected salary for a typical Psychiatrist in the United States is $161,710.

The source for this is CNN Money

This basic market pricing report was prepared using their Certified Compensation Professionals' analysis of survey data collected from thousands of HR departments at employers of all sizes, industries and geographies.

20

Family Practice

Vandana Panda Goyle

INTRODUCTION

Family practice physicians have as their primary commitment the provision of patient-centered care which is bio-psycho-social-spiritual in nature. Family physicians receive 3 years of residency training, they must pass a certifying examination called the ABFP (American Board of Family Practice) a one day exam featuring MCQs to be certified to work anywhere in the US.

After their training is completed, residents can provide the full spectrum of care to their patients, including family-centered prenatal and delivery care, GYN services, adult and child preventive services managing current and chronic illnesses and teaching patients how to prevent or reduce the likelihood of further illness. In other words, family practice provides continuity of care and preventive services to patients of all ages, sexes, inclusive of medical, surgical, obstetric, pediatric and geriatric addressing the needs of the whole person—biologic, psychological/social and spiritual concerns. In doing so, a family practice physician may provide the service directly or coordinate and co-manage the care with an appropriate specialist, with another partner in the group, a counselor, or another community resource.

It can be very much compared with specialty in Community Medicine / PSM in India which mainly takes care of the primary health care plus out-patient services in metro and rural parts of the country.

COMPETITIVENESS OF SPECIALTY

Non-competitive specialty

Applying to programs—individualising curriculum vitae and personal statement

Applications are processed electronically through ERAS (www.myeras.com).

You can apply to as any specialties as you like and an unlimited number of programs, bearing in mind that costs increase with each additional program or specialty applied for (first 10 programs being free).

In addition to your application form, programs request up to four letters of recommendation, a personal statement, a dean's letter and medical school transcripts.

Competition and selection criteria vary widely between programs and specialties. Most surgical specialties are highly competitive and Internal medicine and family medicine are the least competitive. Programs are divided into those that are university based, community based or affiliated to university.

Your graduation year from medical school is incredibly important but few will tell you this.

USMLE scores allow program directors to compare you with American graduates and are Crucial!!, especially Step 1 As a rough guide, for family practice or internal medicine, a passing score can be enough, for general surgery your score should be around 85 to 90 plus experience or Observership in US, and for the most competitive specialties, scores above 95 are required. Letters of recommendations are key. Getting one from and American physician or a renowned specialist is ideal. This is where US experience comes in handy! Once the interview is over and your bank account drained, you will have to wait patiently for the selection process, know as Match, which takes place around march. If you are successful... Congratulations!

RANK ORDER LIST

This is very straightforward. Rank as per your preference. Do not get influenced by the rumor that inevitably floats around every year advising candidates to rank programs based on the probability of the program picking you. Rank every program that you interview at even if you have too many interviews.

DURING RESIDENCY IN YOUR SPECIALTY

Residents rotate through the Departments of Ob/Gyn, Internal medicine, Surgery over the course of their training. In addition, residents rotate with community physicians representing a range of specialties such as surgery, pulmonology, radiology, ophthalmology and neurology.

This includes making ward rounds and medically managing patients who have been admitted to the hospital from the community. Residents usually see their inpatients before office hours in the morning. Additionally, you can choose to do rotations in special interest areas, such as complementary medicine, sports medicine, radiology, geriatrics wards and others. All rotations are well structured and very much geared towards family practice.

Usually the 36 months duration for residency is divided into monthly rotations

	PG Y-1	PGY-2	PGY-3
Family medicine	4.0	2.0	2.0
Cardiology	1.0		
Critical care	1.0		
Emergency medicine	1.0		
Surgery	2.0		
Obstetrics	1.0	1.0	
Pediatrics	2.0	2.0	
Gynecology		1.0	
Orthopedics		1.0	
Rural medicine		1.0	
ENT		0.5	
Ophthalmology		0.5	
Radiology		0.5	
Urology		0.5	
Elective		2.0	4.0
Psychiatry			1.0
Community medicine			1.0
Dermatology			1.0
Internal medicine			2.0
Neurology			1.0

SALARY PROFILES AND LIFESTYLE ISSUES

Residents work an average of eighty hours a week. A typical day starts at 5:30 am and finishes at around 6 pm unless you are on call. Salaries vary, ranging from $ 35000 to $ 45,000 depending on the program and the place. Depending on where you are living, this just about covers expenses.

I will give you a description of what Texas tech is offering, you can make an estimate.

Base/Salary	Relocation	Total
PGY-1 $38,666	$5000	$43,666
PGY-2 $39,927	$2,500	$42,427
PGY-3 $41,188		$41,188

They offer additional perks like book allowance, health, life and dental insurance for resident and immediate family, disability insurance, malpractice insurance, pagers, and meal tickets. List is long!

The average annual salary for the family physician in practice is $ 145000. In rural areas, family physicians with years of experience might earn up to $ 300000.

Obstetrics and Gynecology

Baraa Allaf M

INTRODUCTION

Training consists of a minimum of four years of ACGME—accredited clinically oriented graduate medical education of which three years must be focused on reproductive health care and ambulatory primary health care for women including health maintenance, disease prevention, diagnosis, treatment, consultation and referral. There were 254 obstetrics/gynecology residency programs accredited by the ACGME for 2005/2006 offering 1,154 categorical residency training positions available to the US seniors.

Ob/Gyn is not an "easy" match but it is getting less hard than 10 years ago. In the US popular/well paying specialties go in cycles, take anesthesia: for a long time it was just an average specialty, then no one was going into it... then the reimbursements went through the roof, now it's one of the most competitive/desirable specialties (if you like that sort of thing).

So think about Obs/Gyn. Right now there has been a slow decline over the past six years, in both numbers and percentage of graduates pursuing training in obstetrics and gynecology. Now more spots go unfilled than 10 years ago. More and more people aren't doing deliveries. So think about what will happen to demand! **The IMGs are getting in at the perfect time**. And as for malpractice, the system will implode shortly, it's not sustainable. There's going to be fewer and fewer OB's, then there will be high profile cases of things gone wrong because of OB shortages, and they'll change the laws. It'll be 4-7 years before we finish residency/fellowship, things will change by then and you'll be the only ones standing and able to reap a fantastic job market.

COMPETITIVENESS OF SPECIALTY

Since 2003, interest in obstetrics/gynecology residency positions has been increasing. 98 per cent of these positions were filled this year, 72 per cent by US medical school seniors (up from 68 per cent three years ago). Resource www.NRMP.org.

	2002	2003	2004	2005	2006
Offered Positions	1138	1151	1142	1144	1154
% Filled by AMG's	74.7	68.3	65.1	67.5	72.4
AMG's Matched	850	786	743	772	835
AMG's Unmatched*	20	22	32	47	73
IMG's Matched	217	264	323	311	295
Unfilled Position	71	101	76	61	24

*Among US seniors who ranked only obstetrics and gynecology programs.

The Scale of the Competitiveness:

Ob/Gyn	IM/Pediatrics	Categorical General Surgery
2006 : Intermediate	2006 : Low	2006 : High
2005 : Intermediate	2005 : Low	2005 : High
2004 : Low	2004 : Low	2004 : High
2003 : Low	2003 : Low	2003 : High

APPLYING TO PROGRAMS—INDIVIDUALISING CURRICULUM VITAE AND PERSONAL STATEMENT

During my interviews I found several important factors to have successful Ob/Gyn Match:
- Connection
- Personality is the most important factor in the Ob/Gyn match
- USCE, it is difficult to find elective or observer in the Ob/Gyn, but elective in IM or Surgery is OK
- Very high scores
- University-based programs prefer **fresh grad**
- Strong LOR's especially from US doctors
- Personal statement
- Researches
- Publications
- 1 year prelim surgery makes you a strong candidate

- Ob/Gyn residency in you home country is positive if you are applying to community-based program.

PERSONAL STATEMENT

A wide variety of issues may be raised in your personal statement, including:
- Why are you selecting a particular specialty, or why do you feel particularly well-suited for the specialty to which you are applying?
- What are you looking for in a residency training program?
- At this point in time, what long-range career plans are you considering after your residency training?
- What are your research accomplishments, publications, and/or awards that may have resulted in special recognition from the academic community?
- An autobiographical sketch summarizing your undergraduate years, family, etc., especially they have had a strong impact on your career choice.
- Extracurricular activities, especially if they are not related to the study or practice of medicine.
- Unusual adventures, travel, experience, or outside interests.

Guidelines for Soliciting Letters of Recommendation

- Most programs require a letter from the Ob/Gyn department chair.
- Others should be written by faculty members who know you well, who have worked with you, and who can comment in detail on your personal and professional qualities. These faculty members do not necessarily have to be obstetrician—gynecologists.
- The higher ranking the faculty member who writes the letter, the better. It is helpful, but not absolutely essential, if the person writing the letter is known at the institutions to which you are applying.
- It is much better if you have recommendation letter from faculty members in the US if you did electives under their supervision. For me I sent a letter from the Ob/Gyn department chair in University of Aleppo and two letters from the faculty members in Baylor College of Medicine, Houston. I got it at the end of my internal medicine electives and one letter from the surgery department chair in the Texas Heart Institute.
  — It becomes increasingly important for the FMG to obtain constructive letters of recommendation from the US sources, which might be more easily interpreted by US program directors.

Obstetrics and Gynecology

Friendly IMGs Ob/Gyn residency programs which participated in the 2005-2006 match:

Most of the IMGs friendly programs sponsor **J1 Visa only** especially the University-based programs. The match in the Ob/Gyn at University-based residency program is much more difficult than community-based one. The J1 waiver in Ob/Gyn is available in more than 30 states and is not that difficult.

ALABAMA

- University of South Alabama.

ARIZONA

- Good Samaritan Regional Medical Center.

CONNECTICUT

- Bridgeport Hospital Program.

CALIFORNIA

- Los Angeles County and University of Southern California Program.

ILLINOIS

1. Mount Sinai Hospital Medical Center of Chicago
2. University of Illinois College of Medicine at Peoria Program
3. Southern Illinois University
4. St Francis Hospital of Evanston
5. Saint Joseph Hospital Program
6. Advocate Illinois Masonic Medical Center Program
7. Mercy Hospital and Medical Center Program.

FLORIDA

1. University of Miami-Jackson Memorial Medical Center Program.
2. Orlando Regional Healthcare System Program.

GEORGIA

- Atlanta Medical Center Program

INDIANA

- Indiana University

MASSACHUSETTS

- Baystate Medical Center Program.

MICHIGAN

1. North Oakland Medical Centers
2. William Beaumont Hospital
3. Grand Rapids Medical Education and Research Center
4. Oakwood Hospital Ob/Gyn Residency Program
5. St John Hospital and Medical Center Program
6. Wayne State University/Detroit Medical Center Program
7. Hurley Medical Center/Michigan State University Program
8. Henry Ford Hospital Program
9. Synergy Medical Education Alliance.

NEW YORK

1. Flushing Hospital Medical Center
2. The State University of New York at Buffalo
3. Lenox Hill Hospital
4. St Luke's-Roosevelt Hospital Center
5. Rochester General Hospital
6. Maimonides Medical Center Program
7. Long Island College Hospital Program
8. Lutheran Medical Center Program
9. North Shore University Hospital/NYU School of Medicine Program
10. New York Methodist Hospital Categorical Program
11. Staten Island University Hospital Program
12. SUNY Downstate Medical Center at Brooklyn Program
13. Jamaica Hospital Program.

NEW JERSEY

1. St Barnabas Medical Center Program
2. St Joseph's Regional Medical Center Residency Program.

NORTH CAROLINA

- Pitt County Memorial Hospital/East Carolina University.

OHIO

1. Good Samaritan Hospital.

2. Medical University of Ohio at Toledo Program
3. Case Western Reserve University (Metro Health)
4. Aultman Hospital/NEOUCOM Program.

PENNSYLVANIA

1. Temple University, Philadelphia
2. Lehigh Valley Hospital/Pennsylvania State University
3. Lankenau Hospital
4. Abington Memorial Hospital Program
5. Geisinger Health System
6. Allegheny General Hospital Program
7. Albert Einstein Medical Center
8. Crozer-Chester Medical Center Program
9. Reading Hospital and Medical Center Program.

SOUTH CAROLINA

- Palmetto Health Richland Hospital—University of South Carolina School of Medicine Program

VIRGINIA

- Carilion Health System

WASHINGTON

- Washington Hospital Center Program

WEST VIRGINIA

- West Virginia University (Charleston Division) Program

INTERVIEWING IN YOUR SPECIALTY

Guidelines for Ob/Gyn Residency Interviews

As an interviewee, you are primarily a salesperson. The product you are selling is yourself, and the assets of the product consist of your experience, skills, knowledge, and personality. You communicate your experience and skills in your resume, but your personality come across in the interview. Do not underestimate the impact of the interview. It can open or close the door for you.

The invitation to schedule an interview is a clear indication that you are competitive for the residency program. However, most programs will interview about 10 candidates for every available position. Therefore, prepare carefully for each interview. Use the interview as an opportunity to demonstrate that you are a mature, articulate, and affable individual who has developed realistic, clearly defined career goals. The following guidelines should be helpful to you as you begin this process.

- Be consistently respectful and courteous to the administrative staffing who schedule your interview. A negative comment from an offended staff member can quickly sabotage an otherwise excellent application.
- Schedule your interviews carefully. Be aware of the dangers of inclement weather in certain states during the months of December and January.
- During the actual interview, the most important rule is: relax and be you self.
- Be animated and attentive through the interview and show excitement and interest in being there. **Learn and remember the names of the people who interview you.**
- Be certain that you have several questions to pose to each faculty member and resident with whom you interview. Do not hesitate to ask the same questions of different interviewers. Do not be timid in asking pointed, pertinent questions of the people you meet, but avoid confrontation.
- Watch your body language: how you sit, how you stand, where you put your hands. Eye contact is very important. Have a firm handshake. Try your best to avoid an appearance of indifference or fatigue, particularly at the end of the day.
- Do your homework. Have some knowledge of the program you are visiting and be able to explain why you choose to apply to that institution.
- Develop a list of prepared questions to ask the residents and faculty members. For example
  — How have former residents performed on the CREOG In-Service Training Examination and the written and oral board examinations?
  — How have residents from the program fared when applying for fellowship training?
  — Do all members of the faculty participate actively in teaching the residents?
  — Does the department require that a research project be completed during residency training?
  — What type of administrative and laboratory support is available for resident research projects?
  — Is a night float system in operation?
- Be prepared to answer the following questions that faculty members may pose to you:

- How did you become interested in the specific discipline of obstetrics and gynecology? This question is very important, I answered it in all my interviews.
- What are your plans for the future, i.e. private practice, fellowship training, academic, and research?
- What is your attitude toward abortion? Answer this question forthrightly.
- I see that you have excellent medical achievements in your home country how will you maintain the same level in the US and will not affected by the American lifestyle?
* Throughout the interview, be on your best behavior. Avoid jokes. Avoid assuming too great a familiarity with the residents. Avoid overly casual comments. Avoid any appearance of impropriety.
* **Be humble**. Avoid any trace of arrogance.
* If you decide to cancel an interview, be certain to notify the program director's office by telephone as far in advance of the interview as possible. Do not rely on voice recorders or email. Failure to provide timely notice is an extremely discourteous act, which reflects badly on you and your school. It denies another applicant the opportunity for an interview and inconveniences faculty members and administrators who have set aside time to meet with you.

Evaluate a Specific Residency Program?

Factors to be weighed in selecting a residency program are varied and highly dependent on individual interests. Following are some things to consider when evaluating a residency program:

* Commitment to education (e.g. number of formal teaching conferences, implementation of a structured 4-year curriculum).
* Large versus small, a larger program will give you less work hours and more call coverage and usually are more family friendly.
* University center versus community hospital.
* Ratio of full-time teaching faculty to residents.
* Emphasis on subspecialty education (gynecologic oncology, reproductive endocrinology, maternal—fetal medicine, and urogynecology) versus private practice or primary care.
* Quality of staff/resident and upper-level resident/lower-level resident interpersonal relationships.
* Availability of adequate surgical training in both gynecologic and obstetric procedures (whether you do 500 or 1,000 deliveries does not make much

difference, but if you only get to do three vaginal hysterectomies, it will make a huge difference in your ability to practice independently after graduation from residency).
- Variety of training options offered in the program, e.g. operative laparoscopy and laser surgery, obstetric and endovaginal ultrasonography, and genetics
- Stability and status of the program.
- Degree of change in department staff and leadership over time.
- Number of fellowships obtained by graduates.
- Requirements of the call schedule, particularly the coverage at affiliated hospital.
- Availability of research opportunities and specialized facilities.
- Availability of funds to attend extramural postgraduate courses and present papers at scientific meetings.
    — Keep in mind that every program has different strengths as well as weaknesses, and that there's always room for improvement at every program.

RANK ORDER LIST

Preparing Your Final Match List

- Do not rank any program in which you absolutely would not like to train. However, do not exclude a good program just because of its geographic location. Look for a program that will give you a good education. Do not simply look for a "great place to live." Remember that residency is **only 4 years**.
- Rank programs entirely according to your preferences. Follow your feelings. Do not attempt to guess how programs will rank you or to negotiate arrangements outside of the match.
- Most importantly, remember that the match process is intended to be fair and to produce a "good fit" for both program and applicant. Trust in the essential fairness of the process.
    — I suggest that your number one priority be a strong training experience in an environment where you can be happy and thrive!

The Match Day

Do not be disappointed with your match if you did not match in your first choices. Let's look at the significant upside:
1. You matched, which is much better than the alternative, especially when you consider the dearth of spots.

2. You are going to be in the field of your choice, a goal you have had for most likely a good amount of time.
3. Ultimately, you determine how good of a physician you will be, not your program. Just because you are not training at Hopkins does not mean that you cannot be a fantastic, exceptional physician. Read, read and read, that is what separates the exceptional physicians from the good ones.

Programs lie to applicants just as applicants lie to programs, certainly, I am not the first person to tell you. Being told 'you would make a great addition to our program', 'please consider us when formulating your rank list' are phrases tossed around by programs to ensure that they have an adequate number of people interested.

DURING RESIDENCY IN YOUR SPECIALTY

During Ob/Gyn Residency

Residency training in obstetrics and gynecology is four years in duration. Rotations during these four years will usually be divided between obstetrics, gynecology, gynecologic oncology, reproductive endocrinology, and ultrasonography. Under guidelines established by the Residency Review Committee for Obstetrics and Gynecology, specific educational experiences for the primary and preventive care role of physicians must occupy the equivalent of at least 6 months of the 4 years of residency and may be addressed in any of the 4 years. The primary care rotations will emphasize ambulatory care and will require knowledge and skills in the areas of health maintenance, disease prevention, risk assessment, counseling, and the use of consultants and community resources. These rotations typically include family medicine, internal medicine, emergency medicine, geriatrics, and continuity care clinics.

The rotations and your responsibilities during the residency are somewhat similar in all programs but there are some differences between them depending on the type of the program, university-based or community-based, the facilities and the size of your program. But in general, the rotations and the responsibilities should be as this order.

PGY-1

During your first year you will spend the majority of the year on the obstetric service. And will experience how to triage all full-term and previable patients, perform all full-term vaginal deliveries in addition to primary cesarean sections, and manage the entire low-risk labor wing.

You will also spend 2-3 months on the gynecology service, performing all minor cases, and assisting on major cases. Most of the programs will include also 1-month rotations in the breast surgery, family medicine, and emergency medicine. Some programs may include 1 month rotations in the Ultrasound and Genetics.

PGY-2

In the second year you will be responsible for the management of all high-risk patients in conjunction with the PGY-3 resident. This includes all patients with premature labor, all medical/obstetrical problems, running the antepartum service, managing all inpatients, participating in consultations, and presenting all patients to the obstetrical team for the weekly diabetic and high-risk clinics.

You will spend time on the gynecology service where you will primarily cover outpatient cases consisting of diagnostic and operative hysteroscopies, diagnostic and operative laparoscopies, and tubal ligations. And you will occasionally get to be the first assistant for major cases, the primary objective to be the second assistant for major abdominal and vaginal cases in preparation for your duties of being a PGY-3.

There is also a rotation through the geriatrics department, the HIV pregnancy clinic, psychology, and office urodynamics. Some programs offer a 1 month for research in this year.

PGY-3

You will be responsible for the entire labor and delivery ward, deciding which patients require admission, managing the labor of all low-risk and high risk patients, and operating mostly on benign and malignant abdominal cases. Complex laparoscopy and vaginal surgery are usually included in the 3rd year's experience.

2 months usually included in this year for maternal-fetal medicine rotation and also a 1-month rotation in reproductive endocrinology and an outpatient rotation in internal medicine. In addition to these responsibilities, it is during this year in which your research projects are presented.

PGY-4

The 4th year of the Ob/Gyn residency is a year in which you can hone the skills thus far acquired. A huge emphasis is placed on educating and supervising the junior residents, conducting morning teaching rounds, administrative management, organizing daily lectures, patient care, and gynecologic surgery.

Much time will be spent on the gynecologic service where you will refine your skills and master complex abdominal, laparoscopic, and vaginal surgery, including pelvic reconstruction, with the remaining time spent on the obstetric service.

Some programs offer 1-week to participate in a nation-wide educational conference in your final year.

At the end of your residency the typical experience should be as follows considering you in a good program.

> **Gynecology**

	Primary Surgeon	*Assistant*
Abdominal Hysterectomy	117	55
Vaginal Hysterectomy	41	38
Surgery for Urinary Incontinence	36	55
Operative Laparoscopy	63	29
Hysteroscopy	33	8
Surgical Sterilization	113	45

> **Obstetric**

	Primary Surgeon	*Assistant*
Spontaneous Delivery	275	29
Forceps Delivery	33	3
Cesarean Delivery	196	91
Multifetal Vaginal Deliveries	18	3

Residents are required to take the Council on Resident Education in Ob/Gyn (CREOG) in-training Examination which is given on the third Saturday of January every year. An additional day for the examination as approved by CREOG is provided to the residents to avoid the resident being post-call or on-call during the examination. The exam is given with the security policy of CREOG. This exam is for preparing you for the written boards and to define your weakness area. The CREOG is broken down in Ob, Gyn, REI, Gyn/Onc, preventative and Primary Care, Ethics, Diagnostic Testing, etc...

Recommended textbooks to be read during the residency and for preparing to the board exam:

— Williams Obstetrics, 22nd edition
— Comprehensive Gynecology, 4th edition
— Harrison's Manual of Medicine, 16th edition
— John's Hopkins Manual of Ob/Gyn, 2nd edition
— Te linde's operative Gyn, 9th edition
— Leon Speroff REI, 7th edition
— Drogenmuller Gyn
— Hoskins ONC
— Cecils IM
— Novak's Gynecology, 12th edition
— Ob/Gyn Secrets, 3rd edition
— Essentials of Obstetrics and Gynecology, 4th edition

Factors that go into making you a good resident
1. Always listen to your upper levels/staff.
2. Never be argumentative (especially at rounds or when given direct orders).
3. Know every detail about your patients (cannot be stressed enough).
4. Be a patient advocate.
5. Always be courteous to your support staff (clerks, nurses, techs, etc).
6. By all means avoid the New MD syndrome ("I'm the Doctor, so just do what I say"). You will be second guessed a lot as an intern, and for the most part you will be wrong.
7. Don't be afraid to say "I don't know" (you are an intern; you are not expected to know all the answers). However, do follow all "I don't know" with "Ill" find out by tomorrow".
8. Always complain UP the chain of command, not down (it never looks professional when you complain to the students).
9. Guide the students in the right direction and make sure they know how to present to the upper levels/staff.
10. Answer your pages on time.
11. Never demean or yell at your consultants (you are just as ignorant about their field as they are about yours).
12. Do everything in your power to help expedite labs, or turnover and path reports, etc. (especially applicable at university-based hospitals).
13. Always take time to chat with your patients about something unrelated to their medical problems.
14. Follow all staff commands with "Yes, sir/maam" and "get on it" immediately.
15. When in doubt, ask an upper level.

16. When overwhelmed, ask an upper level.
17. When in need of a drink, ask an upper level.
18. Sleep, eat, and read when you can.
19. Don't be afraid to ask your nurses/scrub techs for advice (many of them have been doing this longer than most residents and even staff).
20. When things are slow, get to know your nurses (many of them will have great stories about your staff when they were residents).
21. Keep up with your reading (5-10 pages/weeknight will keep you more than updated).
22. Never leave the clinic or the hospital until the whole team is done (one for all and all for one).
23. Smile... nobody likes a frown.
24. Remember, everybody above you has gone through the same experience, if not worse (for those that worked in the pre-80 hour work week days). So don't expect any special treatment.
25. Be flexible and creative.
26. Work with your classmates as a team. Do favors for each other and don't be obsessed with who worked more than whom.
27. And lastly, come to the realization that you will make mistakes and make sure that you learn from them!

SPECIALISATION AFTER RESIDENCY

After your 4 years training now you are ready to shoulder your way in several directions that depend on your goals, motivation and Visa status. End up working in private clinic with group, hospital, Academic attending, researcher or doing Fellowship.

Private Practice

Great flexibility exists within this traditional framework. Depending upon the number of partners and nature of specific practice requirements, time can be made available for family and personal needs. Many practices build in a day off each week. Private practice usually offers the widest latitude in selecting a lifestyle or practice mode suited to an individual's specific needs. Among other factors that add to the "satisfaction index" achieved by obstetrician—gynecologists are the long-term relationships with patients, the opportunity to practice preventive medicine, and the challenge of providing a diversity of health care that encompasses a wide spectrum.

Academics

Ten per cent of all board-certified obstetrician-gynecologists are full-time medical school faculty members, many of whom are certified in the subspecialties of gynecologic oncology, maternal-fetal medicine, or reproductive endocrinology. Responsibilities of full-time faculty members include (1) teaching of medical students and house staff, (2) direct patient care, (3) research, and (4) administration.

A key motivation for many physicians in academic medicine is the opportunity for research. The orientation of the studies may be either basic science or clinical medicine.

Academic medicine is a unique discipline with its own standard of rewards that differentiates it from private practice. Financial rewards tend to be less, although they are more competitive now than they were previously.

Subspecialty/Fellowship Training in Obstetrics/Gynecology

There are 4 subspecialties certified by ABOG. When I say certified I mean recognized as a subspecialty with board certification. You will find other so-called subspecialties such as 'adolescent gynecology' and laparoscopy which aren't recognized (yet).

- Ob/Gyn subspecialties are pretty competitive even for those who have completed a residency in Ob/Gyn from the states.
- Earlier on there was a myth that MFM is easy to come by as it is high risk obs (and the trend here is to run away from obs right? Anyway, not so anymore. With 60 odd seats even AMG's find it tough to match in MFM.
- Gynecology Oncology and REI are perhaps the most competitive. Ratio of seat to applicants is 1:50. To get a seat I was told one needs to perform superbly as a resident (AMG/IMG alike).
- You need a visa. AMG's find it tough to match in a subspecialty in Ob/Gyn (its still rare for Ob/Gyns to subspecialize and hence very few seats for applicants who are far more than available seats) for an IMG needing a visa, residency is FAR easier than a fellowship in Ob/Gyn.

1. *Maternal-Fetal Medicine*: A wide range of patient care, research and education is encompassed within this subspecialty. Take care of patients with high-risk pregnancies, including diabetes, preterm labor, hypertension, and others.
2. *Reproductive Endocrinology and Infertility*: A lot of the procedures available include artificial insemination, in vitro fertilization, ovulation induction, and on-going work in male factor infertility problems, among others. Endometriosis, uterine fibroids, and menopausal symptoms are additional

areas of expertise. REI is the 'glamorous' subspecialty' hence also very much in demand.
3. *Gynecology Oncology:* Education, prevention and early detection of cancer, including ovarian cancer screening, are an integral part of this subspecialty. In addition to the treatments which include surgery, radiation therapy, chemotherapy, or combinations of these. Gyn-Onc has about 30-32 seats in the whole of the US and hence cut throat competition.
4. *Urogynecology:* It includes all type of pelvic reconstruction surgery. Disorders of the genitourinary system, surgery, cystoscopy, and urodynamics. Has recently changed from a 1 year course to a 3 years course since it was recognized by the ABOG as a bonafide subspecialty.
5. *Other Options:* Focused practice in laparoscopy, pediatric and adolescent gynecology and reproductive genetics. In this rapidly advancing field are offered genetic counseling, management of fetal anomalies, chorionic villus sampling (CVS), early and midtrimester genetic amniocentesis, fetal ultrasound, and in-utero surgery, as well as others tests and procedures.

Going back home

You have option to go back home to practice Ob/Gyn. Here are the positive points.
— Between your family and your friends
— Better life-style
— Low cost living
— No malpractice
— No taxes
— More money

SALARY PROFILES AND LIFESTYLE ISSUES

How much do Obstetrician-Gynecologists (Ob-Gyn) earn in USA?

With about 1/3rd of a billion in population and more than half a million immigrants pouring in each year, looks like it will be green for Ob/Gyn specialist physicians for a long time! Let's see some quick numbers:

Mean start salary	$ 227,000
Median start salary	$ 200,000

After 1-2 years of experience:

Median salary	$ 244,000
Mean salary	$ 284,000

The salary is depending on the type of practice, location and works hours. That is up to you, during the one of my interview, one of the 4th year residents told us that he got job in Illinois with annual start salary of $ 250,000?!!.

The Ob/Gyn lifestyle

Personally, I almost went into Internal Medicine for lifestyle reasons and switched to Ob at the last minute. I know my life will be more difficult in many ways, but I'm so much more interested and passionate about Ob/Gyn, that I *hope* the sacrifice will be worth it. I figure you still have to work 80 hours/week in most fields in medicine (certainly in IM and OB), you might as well love what you are doing with those 80 hours.

It is important that you make your own decision, realizing that parental and family disappointments now will disappear with the future with a happier son or daughter who has fulfilled his or her own goals.

Ultimately this has to be your personal decision. For me, I was willing to sacrifice my lifestyle for a while to go to work every day knowing I was going to love what I do.

Happiness in medicine is where you find it AND where you make it. No specialty is perfect for everyone. But, no specialty is terrible as well. People that talk poorly about other specialties usually either had a single bad experience or use that to try to tarnish the field, they don't know what they are talking about, or they are the types of persons that think that the only good thing on earth is what they themselves are doing. None of these people ever seem to offer good advice... so, be careful what you listen to and avoid taking to heart other's judgments of a field. **Make your own decisions and allow others to do the same.**

Anyway, the Ob/Gyn offers flexible lifestyles, whether you are in a private, group, or academic practice. In the past, being an obstetrician/gynecologist meant a busy lifestyle with hectic call schedules. At present, call groups have been developed to give physicians greater flexibility with on-call days and working hours. You also can choose your scope of practice: part-time, office-only gynecology, hospital inpatient care, large group, academic faculty, or obstetric surgery.

Ob/Gyn is not an "easy" match, and it is going to be harder and harder in front of the closed doors in the UK. Look at the 2006 match statistics. Only 24 seats in the whole of the US remain unfilled, but it is certainly within reach if you work hard. There are a lot of programs out there, some tougher than others, but you will find a very few that you love and that love you. True enthusiasm shows through the application and interview, and it is always well received. There is a lot more to matching than simply your Step scores.

Neurology

Disha Uttam Shah

INTRODUCTION

Neurology is emerging as an IMG friendly specialty in the US. From 2006-2007 onwards, Neurology is moving to ERAS and NRMP, which is good news, as applicants will be able to rank Neurology programs, which are not integrated, along with the preliminary Internal Medicine programs and come to know the results together. This is in contrast to the SFMatch (www.sfmatch.org) for Neurology which was an earlier match than the NRMP. Neurology is a residency in the US to be done after a year of Preliminary Internal Medicine, unlike in India where it is a fellowship to be done after the categorical Internal Medicine Residency. Neurology begins from the year PGY2 and it is of 3 years, thus the duration of residency becomes 4 years including the PGY1 year. Some of the residency programs are integrated, i.e. include the first year of preliminary Internal Medicine (PGY1) while other residency programs do not offer the PGY1 preliminary year which has to be applied for and interviewed for separately. Some residency programs may offer an interview for PGY1 if you apply for Neurology there, but do not guarantee a spot.

COMPETITIVENESS OF SPECIALTY

Neurology is a relatively non-competitive specialty in the United States.

APPLYING TO PROGRAMS—INDIVIDUALISING CURRICULUM VITAE AND PERSONAL STATEMENT

From my experience, I think more than scores, neurology residency programs look for some clinical or research experience in Neurology and obviously graduates with masters or PhD in Neuroscience are given preference. International Medical Graduates interested in pursuing Neurology in the US, should try to do a rotation in Neurology in a hospital or with a privately practicing Neurologist in their home country, and get a recommendation letter documenting the same to enhance their application. The best thing would be to get some US clinical or research experience in Neurology. The personal statement should reflect the person's integrity and also what attracts him/her to Neurology as a specialty. A prepared CV and personal statement can be provided while asking for letters of recommendation from Neurology faculty with whom you do your rotation.

Applying to programs

What programs to apply to depend on the individual's preferences. Programs can be choosen depending on their location and reputation. Another important thing to look for in a Neurology program is the subspecialty representation it has, in terms of the faculty and rotations available. For example, someone interested in pursuing a fellowship in Stroke should find out more about the experience in Stroke that the Neurology residency program offers. The most important factor which matters for IMGs while applying to residency programs is whether that program sponsors visas and whether it is the kind of visa they are looking for. The number of programs to apply also depends on the individual, whether one is looking for integrated programs only or H-1B sponsoring programs only. According to my experience, an international medical graduate should preferably apply to around 30 programs in Neurology and if they have applied to nonintegrated Neurology programs also, then at least around 20 preliminary Internal Medicine programs should be applied to as preliminary positions are very competitive.

Information about neurology residency programs which participated in the 2005-2006 match is as follows—

Integrated Neurology Programs (including PGY1) with no. of positions.

ALABAMA

1. U. Alabama -3 www.uab.edu/neuroresidency
2. U South Alabama-2

ARIZONA

- Mayo Clinic, Scottsdale-3 www.mayo.edu/mgsm/snr.htm

ARKANSAS

- U. Arkansas-4 www.uams.edu/neurology/index.htm

CALIFORNIA

- UC Davis-1 neurology.ucdavis.edu

ILLINOIS

1. Northwestern University-4 or 5 www.neurology.northwestern.edu
2. U of IL-Peoria COM-2 www.uicomp.uic.edu/neurores/
3. Southern Illinois U-2 www.siumed.edu/resaffairs/NEURO.htm

INDIANA

- Indiana U-1 or 2 neurology.medicine.iu.edu/residencyprogram

IOWA

- U Iowa -5 www.uihealthcare.com/depts/med/neurology

KENTUCKY

- U Kentucky-3 www.mc.uky.edu/neurology/

LOUISIANA

1. LSU-Shreveport-3 www.sh.lsuhsc.edu/neurology/
2. Tulane University-3 or 4 www.tmc.tulane.edu/

MICHIGAN

- U Michigan-2 www.med.umich.edu/neuro/

MINNESOTA

- U Minnesota, Mpls-5 www.neurology.umn.edu

MISSOURI

1. U Missouri, Columbia-3 http://neurology.muhealth.org/
2. St. Louis University-4 medschool.slu.edu/departments/neurology/
3. Washington University-8 www.neuro.wustl.edu

NEW YORK

1. Albany Medical College-3 www.amc.edu/gme/neurology_residency.htm
2. SUNY-Buffalo-3 www.thejni.org
3. New York Hosp/Cornell U-6 www.med.cornell.edu/neuro/education/res_prog.html
4. SUNY-StonyBrookMED/NEUR-1or 2 www.hsc.stonybrook.edu/index.cfm?id=144

NORTH CAROLINA

1. U North Carolina-4 neuron.med.unc.edu/neurology/
2. Wake Forest U-4 www.wfubmc.edu

OHIO

1. Cleveland Clinic Found.-7 www.clevelandclinic.org/neurology/education/
2. Med U Ohio-Toledo-2 www.meduohio.edu/depts/neurology

OKLAHOMA

- U Oklahoma, Oklahoma City-3 w3.ouhsc.edu/neuro

OREGON

- Oregon HSU-3 www.ohsu.edu/neurology/residency

PENNSYLVANIA

1. Temple U, Philadelphia-4 www.temple.edu/neuro
2. Jefferson U, Phil-0 or 3 www.jefferson.edu/neurology
3. U Pittsburgh-5 www.neurology.upmc.edu/Residencyneurology.htm
4. U Pennsylvania-2 www.uphs.upenn.edu/neuro/index.html

SOUTH CAROLINA

- Med U South Carolina-4 www.musc.edu/neurology/

TENNESSEE

1. U Tennessee, Memphis-3 or 4 www.utmem.edu/neurology/
2. Vanderbilt University-4 www.mc.vanderbilt.edu/neurology/

TEXAS

- UT Southwestern-1 or 5 neurology.swmed.edu

VIRGINIA

- U Virginia-5
 http://www.healthsystem.virginia.edu/Internet/neurology/training/residency-program.cfm

WASHINGTON

- U Washington-4 or 5 www.neurology.washington.edu

WISCONSIN

- U Wisconsin-2 or 4 www.neurology.wisc.edu

There are many more non-integrated Neurology Programs. Most of the IMG friendly programs sponsor J1 visa.

The residency programs which were **sponsoring H-1B visa** for the 2005-2006 match, i.e. for PGY2 beginning in the year 2007 were as follows. (This information is subjected to change and should be verified with the program).

1. U Alabama
2. Yale University
3. Cleveland Clinic Florida
4. U Florida-Gainesville
5. Emory U, Georgia
6. U Illinois-Peoria COM
7. Tufts/New England MC
8. Wayne State University
9. Mayo Clinic-Rochester
10. U Missouri-Columbia
11. New Jersey Neuroscience Inst
12. Albert Einstein COM
13. New York Hosp/Cornell U
14. AECoM North Shore-LIJ
15. Mount Sinai SoM
16. SUNY-Brooklyn
17. U Cincinnati
18. Cleveland Clinic Foundation
19. Med U Ohio-Toledo
20. Drexel U

21. Temple U-Philadelphia
22. Jefferson U-Philadelphia
23. Med C Wisconsin

Some useful links

>   www.nrmp.org
>   www.neurology.org
>   www.aan.com
>   http://forums.studentdoctor.net/forumdisplay.php?f=48

INTERVIEWING IN YOUR SPECIALTY

The interview

After applying to your desired programs, wait for the interview invitations which may come via regular mail, email or rarely via telephone. As with other specialties, do not schedule the interview at your most desired program first, as it takes a few interviews to warm up and become confident. Interviews in Neurology focus on the applicant's personality as well as on their Curriculum Vitae. Most of the interviews I attended started with a general overview of the residency programs and then individual interviews with a few faculty members and maybe a chief resident. At one of the programs there was a panel interview in which all the applicants were asked the same question at the same time and they had to answer one by one, giving an answer which was different than others. Another interview I attended had 7 interviews with individual faculty members and I was asked medical questions related to Neurology at some places. The key is to remain confident while giving answers and be able to convince the interviewer why you want to go into Neurology.

It is always a good idea to note down points during or after the interview about that program, which you can use later while writing your thank you note to that residency program.

RANK ORDER LIST

Preparing your rank order list

It goes without saying that always rank the programs in the order in which you would like to match. Your interview performance or feedback from the program does not matter. Some criteria can come to play regarding whether the program is integrated, offers desired fellowships etc. depending on what you are looking for.

SPECIALISATION AFTER RESIDENCY

Some fellowships which can be done after Neurology Residency:
- Vascular Neurology (Stroke)
- Movement Disorders
- Epilepsy
- Sleep Medicine
- Behavioral Neurology
- Neuroimmunology (Multiple Sclerosis)
- Neuromuscular disorders
- Neurorehabilitation
- Critical Care Neurology
- Clinical Neurophysiology
- Pain Medicine
- Interventional Neuroradiology
- Neuro-Oncology
- Advanced Clinical Neurology
- AIDS
- Alzheimer's Disease
- Dementia
- Geriatric Neurology
- Headache
- Neuroepidemiology
- Neurogenetics
- Neuroimaging
- Neuroophthalmology
- Neurootology
- Neuropathology
- Neuropharmacology
- Neurorehabilitation
- Neurovirology
- Spine

SALARY PROFILES AND LIFESTYLE ISSUES

The median expected salary for a typical Physician—Neurology in the United States is $177,734.

Surgery

Pragatheeswar Thirunavukkarasu

INTRODUCTION

Surgery in the United States. This sentence may ring bells in the brains of many students, but the truth is that most of those rings are due to sheer ignorance. All the golden rules for a good application like good scores and good curriculum vitae hold good for surgery too, but nevertheless, there is a whole lot of information that IMGs need to know about surgical specialties in the USA. That is a whole new world!

Many IMGs don't apply for surgical specialties as much as they do for medical specialties.

Some of the reasons that are often given for this are as follows:
1. Surgical specialties are competitive.
2. IMGs are given second preference to USMGs during residency selection process in surgical specialties.
3. Surgical residents have bad and long work hours.
4. Surgical residencies take longer time to finish.
5. Surgical residencies are malignant and exploitative of the IMGs.
6. Surgery is losing its charm and the trend will continue so.

While most of the above statements may sound reasonable, they are hardly the full truth. Before we venture to explore how surgical specialties differ from other specialties, we need to analyze the truth behind several opinions about surgical specialties that are widely prevalent among IMGs. Let's do it one by one.

COMPETITIVENESS OF SPECIALTY

Preliminary Surgery, one year is non-competitive whereas categorical General Surgery, five years is very competitive. As International Medical Graduates, one has to do preliminary surgery for a few years before getting into Categorical General surgery.

Yes. Absolutely true. No doubt. All surgical specialties are very competitive. One of popular residency guides in the market classified all possible specialties into 5 categories, based on the level of competitiveness and difficultness of entering into it. Category I is the easiest and Category V is supposed to be the toughest. In this classification, Category V, which is the most difficult, is constituted by 3 specialties namely, Orthopedic Surgery, Plastic Surgery and Urology. Category IV, which is second in difficulty only to Category V specialties, is composed of General Surgery, Otorhinolaryngology, Neurosurgery and other surgical specialties. It is obvious that almost all surgical specialties are very competitive.

But the above classification is not absolute and evergreen. The ranking of the specialties based on their competitiveness varies from match to match, from place to place and from institution to institution. For example, Family medicine or neurology residencies (less competitive specialties) in Harvard or Ivy League universities are much more competitive than General Surgery in a less than average residency program in a suburb or rural area in New Mexico.

And, depending upon the current and floating health policies, insurance reimbursement policies and malpractice coverage policies, the importance and competitiveness of certain specialties may rise and fall with time and this fluctuation may be drastic and unexpected enough to raise eyebrows. The best example is Anesthesia. There was a time when anesthesia program directors couldn't even hire rats to enter their residencies but out of the blue, anesthesia is one of the 'hot' specialties during the past few years.

But all said and done, surgery continues to be competitive regardless of several factors that have been affecting its dynamics. One of the most important of such factors is the Work hour limitations. Surgery residencies are notorious for being very laborious, tiring and draining, both physically and mentally. Surgical residents often complain of long work hours, even as long as 110 to 115 hours per week. There were increasing reports of marital discord, loss of quality of life outside the hospital, lack of time for academic activities and teaching and diminishing morale among the surgical community in the USA, which is when Americans, who revere lifestyle as an important attribute to good quality of life, began to look away from surgery as a career choice. It is at this time, that surgical specialties, especially general surgery became less competitive among USMGs, thereby creating room for IMGs. This can be called the honeymoon period for IMGs aspiring to become surgeons in the USA.

But like all honeymoons, this was also shortlived. The issue of increasing exploitation of surgical residents and downhill course of general surgery gained importance with time until the popular, controversial and currently applicable "80 hour work rule" was imposed. According to this rule, all residents irrespective of their specialties should stay in the hospital for no longer than 80 hours per week. The rule also entails the necessity of a 24 hours completely duty free period every week.

After the imposition of this rule, surgical residents had better lives both inside and outside the hospital. Surgery began to regain its lost glory of competitiveness to so much that it has less unfilled positions than even orthopedic surgery during the 2006 match.

APPLYING TO PROGRAMS—INDIVIDUALISING CURRICULUM VITAE AND PERSONAL STATEMENT

Now we shall begin to discuss step by step the facts about entering surgical specialties. Most of the information presented here is more consistent with general surgery, since it is the most sought after surgical specialty by IMGs.

Making the decision

Making the decision to pick the knife instead of the pen will make a sea of difference in your life. It is necessary for each student to discriminate the lifestyle between physicians and surgeons. Explaining the difference in detail is beyond the scope of this book. Making the decision to specialize in surgery is separate and discrete from the decision to do it in the USA.

Deciding to do surgery is tougher and requires more time and analysis than deciding to enter the USA. However, deciding to do surgery in the USA is a very difficult decision to make. This is so, because surgery in the USA is not a straightforward option for the IMGs. IMGs have to do a lot of 'foreplay' before even getting into the actual game.

To decide to do surgery in the USA, we need to:
a. Make the decision as early as possible.
b. Be genuinely interested and attracted and excited to be a surgeon (or else, it might feel like in hell to work with surgeons).
c. Be very committed to the purpose of surgery.
d. Be prepared for failure as it is bound to happen too many times, given the less number of seats available for IMGs and the disproportionately large number of eligible students applying for it.

e. Have alternate plans and backups in case failure occurs.
f. Be prepared to spend years off just trying to get into the actual residency.
g. Be prepared for difficult and hard years of training for a minimum of 5-7 years.
h. Be prepared for a difficult life even during the later years of practice to come.
i. Be prepared to sacrifice personal and family interests at least to some extent.
j. Ensure that your spouse and family understand the nature and quality of your work.
k. Understand the dynamics of income in surgery like the reimbursement policies, malpractice insurance, referral services, etc.
l. Be ready to invest money on instruments and theaters in case you have decided to start your own health care setup, in case you want to return to India.

IMGs are given second preference to USMGs during residency selection process in surgical specialties.

This is also true though it may not be the whole truth. USMGs are usually preferred to IMGs by program directors in general and there are several studies to support this statement. But this preference cannot be fully explained by racial and discriminative factors alone. The problem is deeper than it appears.

IMGs are a heterogeneous group. They may be from India, Pakistan, South America, China, Europe, Middle East, etc. The program directors are little aware of what is the standard and type of medical education in all of these countries. So they just want to play it safe by hiring a candidate who is trained in and by a system that they are aware of.

It is important to note that the discrimination is not based on whether the applicant is a US citizen or not. It is only based on whether he was a medical graduate in the US or not. For example, a foreign national who did his medical education in the USA is a USMG, who will be clearly preferred to a US citizen who was trained abroad (technically an IMG).

Some other reasons why IMGs are not preferred are as follows:
a. IMGs don't speak English well.
b. IMGs lack communication skills while interacting with American patients.
c. IMGs find it difficult to get along with their fellow American colleagues.
d. IMGs have more background problems.
e. IMGs are not used to working in the American setup, which makes them difficult to train more than American graduates.
f. IMGs are often old and far from graduation making them less malleable for training.

At this juncture, it is important to realize that we, Indians (who think that we are often sincere and hardworking), are not the only people who constitute the IMG population. In fact, we constitute the minority. There are scores of IMGs from Europe, China and South America.

The disadvantage that IMGs suffer because they are IMGs is even higher as we move up the ladder of competitive specialties. In surgical specialties, there is already a surplus of eligible USMGs and hence these programs don't have to take the risk of hiring an IMG for the reasons mentioned above. Furthermore, some program directors are under the pressure from their conscious self and from others to rank USMGs with lesser achievement profiles higher than IMGs with better profiles.

So, it is true that IMGs are disadvantaged and it is truer in competitive specialties like surgical specialties.

But it is untrue that program directors are totally averse to hiring an IMG. They do take IMGs, only when they are exceptional. So, exceptional IMGs don't often feel discriminated but the average IMG does. There are also some programs which have committed themselves to encouraging ethnic diversity and hence take IMGs on a regular basis.

But the bottomline is, more is expected out of an IMG than from a USMG in the same platform.

RANK ORDER LIST

This is very straightforward. Rank as per your preference. Do not get influenced by the rumor that inevitably floats around every year advising candidates to rank programs based on the probability of the program picking you. Rank every program that you interview at even if you have too many interviews.

DURING RESIDENCY IN YOUR SPECIALTY

Surgery—Preliminary and Categorical

There are 2 types of spots in surgery that are available for the match. They are 'preliminary' and 'categorical'.

When a candidate is hired at the PGY1 level as a 'categorical', it means that he is selected once and for all for the next required number of years required to complete his entire residency. In other words, the progression to the next consecutive year (PGY2) and then to the next forthcoming years (PGY3, 4, 5) is guaranteed and without bottlenecks, as far as the resident satisfies the usual requirements during his training.

On the contrary, when a candidate is hired at the PGY1 level as a 'preliminary', it means he is selected for that academic year alone. He has to apply afresh for the next year. He is not guaranteed a position in that residency program or elsewhere in the USA for the next year.

Preliminary spots are available in both medicine and surgery. Some specialties like neurology, anesthesia, radiology, etc (which are called advanced positions) require the residents to complete their first year of residency—otherwise called "internship" either in general medicine or general surgery. So these candidates who match for the specialty programs in certain institutions may apply for preliminary spots in other programs. Usually such advanced residency applicants choose to do their preliminary years in general medicine instead of general surgery due to obvious reasons—less workload, more free time, less intensive call schedules, less pressure at work, etc.

Preliminary surgery spots are of 2 types—designated and non-designated. Designated preliminary spots are only for candidates who have already matched for an advanced position. For example, a candidate who is applying for radiology residencies might apply and interview for preliminary surgery spots. He needs to match in both, but his match for the radiology residency is for the year after the next, while the preliminary year is for the immediate next. Only such candidates who are applying for other advanced positions can be filled in the 'designated preliminary spots'. Non-designated preliminary spots are those that are filled by candidates without advanced positions. These candidates are those who weren't good enough to match into categorical surgical positions straightaway and hence are attempting to apply for categorical positions after doing a year or two in preliminary surgery. During these years they might work hard and make their CV more impressive, better by improving the number of publications, getting better letters of recommendation, improving their contacts, etc.

Non-designated preliminary surgery positions are also taken up by candidates who are attempting to enter into other surgical specialties like urology, plastic surgery, orthopedic surgery, otorhinolaryngology, etc. These residencies require one or two years of specialty training, which may not be necessarily completed in the same institution as the final years of residency. So, candidates who are unable to match in the institution of their choice in these specialties may do a year or two or preliminary surgery in some other institutions in non-designated spots, during which time they keep applying for the spots of their choice.

Program directors in surgery may be quite skeptical about IMGs due to reasons discussed above. So, they might want to be sure if the IMG is good and compatible with the program before hiring him for a categorical spot. Their best bet is to hire him for a non-designated preliminary spot and assess him for a year. Later, if the PD finds him good, then he may hire him for a categorical spot.

So, IMGs aiming to enter into surgery often have a brighter chance of entering a non-designated preliminary spot instead of a straight categorical spot. But, there is always a huge portion of uncertainty surrounding this decision to do a preliminary year. The explanation for this is as follows:

For every 1 categorical general surgery spot in an institution, there may be up to 5 preliminary surgery spots in the same institution. Some programs have a definite number of those preliminary spots for designated candidates while others don't have any such preclusion. Therefore, there is more number of non-designated preliminary sports in general surgery than the categorical spots. This means that all those who do preliminary surgery will not enter into categorical positions the next year. Many of them will be dropped out. Often the estimated percentage of preliminary surgery residents who don't end up as categoricals may be as high as 80%.

Also, after completing a preliminary year in general surgery, the candidate may end up as a categorical resident, but not necessarily at the PGY2 level. After assessing the candidate's performance, the program may hire him as categorical at the PGY1 level, in which case he would have to repeat his first year (internship).

This is not a rule. The reasons why preliminary residents are hired at the PGY1 level is are:

a. The program may be hiring all their categorical residents at the PGY1 level and if none of them drops out, there may be no vacancies at the PGY2 for the preliminary candidates to fill.
b. The program may have slightly different rotation schedules for the preliminary interns and categorical interns. So, they might expect the preliminary resident to work again as a PGY1 in order that the candidate has the same schedule as the program's other categorical residents.
c. Some programs might have a policy to do a national search every time a spot opens up at higher levels, instead of filling them with their own preliminary residents. This may be to satisfy all faculty members, some of whom may feel that a better candidate might be available to fill in their vacant spot.

What is very important to understand here is that most IMGs who do preliminary surgery will start their categorical residents as PGY1. It is only often a matter of luck for a prelim PGY2 to enter into a PGY2 straightaway.

Also, preliminary surgery spots are not only available at the PGY1 level, but also at the PGY2 level. So, a preliminary PGY1 may end up as PGY2 instead of being absorbed into the categorical stream. The dynamics become more complicated in this case.

At the end of PGY2 preliminary year, the candidate may be taken as a categorical starting from the PGY1 level, in which case he repeats the first 2 years again. Also, even after completing the PGY2 preliminary year, there is no guarantee that he might become a categorical next year.

Surgical residencies take longer time to finish

This is also true. The internal medicine residency takes 3 years, while all surgical residencies require a minimum of 5 years to complete. In some universities, residents are strongly encouraged to take 1 or 2 off for research, thereby making it a total of 7-9 years. The latter is especially true of general surgical residencies in some top university programs.

This is an important factor for many American medical graduates who have huge student loans and a family to support. For those who want to start a clinical practice as soon as possible and start paying their loans off, surgery is a bad option.

Surgical residencies are malignant and exploitative of the IMGs

The above statement, though is popularly heard in IMG discussions, in my opinion, is an exaggeration of the fact that surgical residents often do more draining and tiring work. When surgical residents don't perform up to the expectations of the faculty, they are often dealt with seriously. This is understandable, because surgeons function as teams and even if one person is a misfit, the morale of the whole team is spoilt. So, a misfit is often dealt with or without much mercy. This may lead to eviction of the resident and the program gets the label of being malignant and exploitative.

But if you are a keen observer, you may notice that no one benefits from a malignant program, neither the faculty nor the residents. But malignancy is unavoidable when the residents and faculty don't match. And more competitive specialties tend to be more intolerant of the deficiencies of their residents, due to their ease of filling up a voided position. But a program with a high drop out is less attractive, even though it may belong to a competitive specialty. So the program director and faculty of competitive residencies avoid hiring an IMG in order to evade the risk of hiring a person who has a larger probability of being a misfit.

Due to such obvious reasons, IMGs experience a lower level of tolerance in surgical residencies.

Surgery is losing its charm and the trend will continue to be so

It is not totally true. Nevertheless, surgery is not a very attractive option for reasons mentioned above. But mostly the argument is that of sour grapes.

SPECIALIZATION AFTER RESIDENCY

SALARY PROFILES AND LIFESTYLE ISSUES

Surgical residents have bad and long work hours:
True. As said above surgical residents often worked more hours than their medical counterparts. But now, after the imposition of the 80-hour-work-rule, this has been no longer a problem. But though it's only 80 hours per week, it's 80 long hours…

Surgical residents have a tighter and more pressure-loaded schedule than medical residents. Moreover, surgeons are generally considered to be a more 'difficult' group of people to interact with and work under. Many USMGs quote this as reason for not looking upon surgery as a career option.

The intention of elaborating on all these aspects is definitely not to discourage IMG surgical aspirants but to make them aware of the risks involved in applying to surgery, lest they should regret the loss of money, effort and most importantly time involved in being preliminary residents, which is nothing but a gamble in the disguise of propping up for the categorical spots.

The annual salary for general surgeons ranges from $ 2, 49, 700 to $ 3, 36, 000.

24

Other Competitive Specialties

Muralikrishna G

LIST OF OTHER SPECIALTIES

Anesthesiology
Dermatology
Emergency Medicine
Neurological Surgery
Orthopaedic Surgery
Transitional Year
Urology
Otolaryngology
Plastic Surgery
Radiation Oncology
Radiology Diagnostic

General rules to get into competitive specialties

- You have to compete with American Medical Graduates.
- May have to compromise on geographic location or quality of program.
- Need high scores on the USMLE and first attempts on all Steps.
- ECFMG certificate and USMLE Step 3 at the time of application.
- Research in particular specialty in the United States, preferably in a top University under a well known researcher with presentations and publications in your name.

- Clinical experience, preferably in the US, also at home country in the specialty for which you are applying.
- Additional degree or fellowship in the specialty you are applying for.
- No visa issues preferably (GC holder or US citizen).
- Personal contacts in the specialty.
- US letters of recommendation—from University hospitals with residency—program, from well known clinician, strong letter, with specific examples and hands-on clinical experience.
- Prior residency in home country or recent graduate (within 3-5 years).

Section Seven
What After the Match?

25

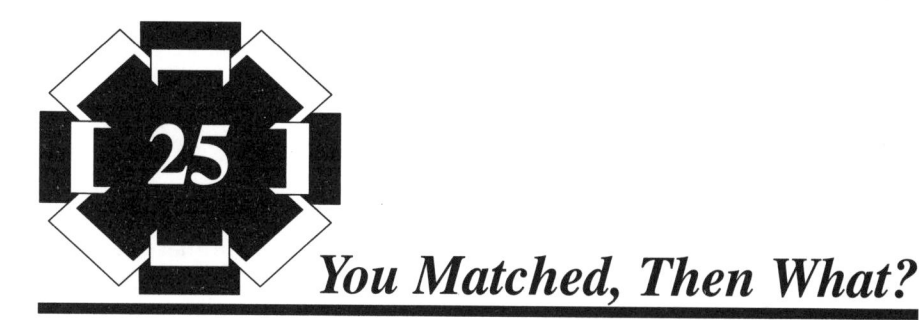

You Matched, Then What?

Archana Bhaskaran

So your dream of long ago has come true at last. This is indeed an achievement. Congratulations. However, there is still one last step before you set foot in your residency program. The following need to be done though not necessarily in the same order.
1. Sign the contract
2. Obtain license to practice medicine
3. File the visa petition
4. Decide on your rotation schedule
5. Complete health requirements
6. Fix visa appointment
7. Prepare for the visa interview
8. Expenditure—postmatch

Every state and residency program has different sets of procedures and the following only give a general overall picture.
1. Once you know where you have matched, email or call the concerned program director to thank them. They will mail the contract to you which needs to be signed on a yearly basis. Therefore, this will be the first of your three. At the same time you will be informed of your duties, benefits including vacation time, salary, etc.
2. Most states in the US require you to have a license to practice medicine. There is also a fee accompanying it which varies from state to state. States like New York do not require a license which saves some valuable time.
3. If you do require a visa, the concerned residency program will file your visa petition at the US Department of Homeland Security. Copies of documents that will be required for the same are:

a. Degree certificate
b. ECFMG certificate
c. Score reports, all Steps
d. Curriculum Vitae
e. Personal Statement
f. Passport

Unless your placement was a prematch it is most likely that premium processing of the visa has to be done to speedup. It costs dollar 1000. Who pays for it, you or the program varies, but even if you do pay for it you can request a waiver after joining residency. At this point you might have to follow your visa with the attorney (Appointed by the Program) Rather than the Program Coordinator. Also you might have to shell out attorney fee which varies widely from one lawyer to another. Be aware of your petition or receipt number which can be used to track the status of your petition at the USCIS website.

4. Some programs like to decide the rotation schedule early for every resident. They can email you with the possible templates from which you can choose (some others want to know only when you will be scheduling your vacation). In such a situation choose depending on the number of and timing of the electives (if you are interested in a subspecialty), vacation slot, etc.

5. We as doctors are fortunate to be familiar with the immunization part as otherwise this is Greek and Latin to non-medical personnel. The diseases which are of public health importance in the US with regard to internationals are.

    a. Tuberculosis—PPD testing/CXR if past history of TB.
    b. Chickenpox-H/O chickenpox/documentation of vaccination or immunity.
    c. MMR-documentation of vaccination or immunity.
    d. Hepatitis B-documentation of vaccination or immunity.
    e. Tetanus vaccination and may be diphtheria too.

    Immunity to b, c, d can be proved by serum titres of the specific antibody. MMR vaccine can be taken in adulthood: 2 doses (2nd dose required as we are foreign nationals) at least 28 days apart. Chickenpox too follows the same schedule. Hepatitis as we all know needs three doses at 0, 1, 6 months.

6. This applies if you are in your home country and need to stamp your visa at the US consulate. Visa appointments are difficult to come by. The usual waiting time can be 2 to 5 months. Since you will need an appointment in a month or so keep checking the availability of dates as new early ones can pop up either due to cancellations or because the consulate releases new slots. If you are going for a J1 Visa, you are eligible to book under emergency

appointments too in contrast to H-1B. For the latter you can mail the consulate and request with your details an early appointment. To book an appointment the petition or receipt number and the HDFC DD number is essential.

7. First get the documents ready for the visa interview. They are:
   a. DS 156, DS 158, Passport, Appointment receipt, Demand drafts
   b. I-797, I-129, LCA
   c. Contract
   d. Letter from the program director stating your employment, salary.
   e. Brochure of the University.
   f. Printout of the NRMP account which displays where you have matched.
   g. All relevant USMLE documents—ECFMG certificate, all score reports, recommendation letters, CV, PS.
   h. Medical degree certificate, score sheets of you MBBS days, any awards or honors. You can also take similar ones from your school.
   i. Financial details, either yours or your parents. This is not required as you are getting a stipend but it is better to be safe than sorry.
   j. Take your itinerary if you have booked your flight tickets.

   Be confident, relaxed and yourself—just like interviews for the residency. Do not show your anxiety and don't be fidgety. Talk slow and clear and answer truthfully.

8. Expenditure postmatch.
   All this is an approximate figure:
   a. License–Dollar 150
   b. Visa fee to US Department of Homeland Security—dollar 200
   c. Premium processing fee—dollar 1000
   d. Attorney fee—dollar 1000 to 2500
   e. Postage fee for sending documents to the US via FedEx (if you are in your homeland)—dollar 150
   f. Flight ticket to the US (if you are in your homeland)—dollar 800
   g. Visa appointment fee—dollar 150
   h. Shopping for setting house in the US—dollar 1000

Section Eight
Miscellaneous

26

Suggested Reading, Website Links, Official Links

Muralikrishna G

APPLYING FOR THE USMLE Step 1, Step 2 CK, and Step 2 CS EXAMS:
FOR MEDICAL STUDENTS: https://iwa2.ecfmg.org/studentoverview.asp
  FOR GRADUATES: https://iwa2.ecfmg.org/gradoverview.asp
APPLYING FOR STEP 3:
  FSMB website: http://www.fsmb.org/usmle_applonline.html
  STATE-SPECIFIC REQUIREMENTS FOR STEP 3: http://www.fsmb.org/usmle_requirementschart.html
APPLYING FOR A VISA:
  VFS-USA: https://www.vfs-usa.co.in/Home.aspx

OFFICIAL WEBSITES

- www.ecfmg.org
- www.usmle.org
- www.sfmatch.org
- www.nbme.org
- www.fsmb.org
- FIND A RESIDENT: http://www.aamc.org/students/findaresident/
- IS THIS PROGRAM ACCREDITED?: http://www.acgme.org/adspublic/
- FORUMS

FOR ALL STEPS

- www.usmle.net
- www.usmleforum.com

- www.prep4usmle.com
- http://forums.studentdoctor.net/

LINKS TO COURSES: ALL STEPS:

http://www.kaplanmedical.com/
http://www.exammaster.com/

STEP 1

ANATOMY

NET ANATOMY: http://www.netanatomy.com/

PATHOLOGY

WEB PATH: http://medstat.med.utah.edu/WebPath/webpath.html

STEP 2 CK

CONRAD FISCHER COURSES: http://www.medicineboardreview.com/main/courseDescription.asp

STEP 2 CS

PASS CSA: http://www.passcsa.com/
USMLEWORLD: http://www.usmleworld.com/

APPLYING TO PROGRAMS

FREIDA: http://www.ama-assn.org/ama/pub/category/2997.html
PROGRAM REVIEWS: www.scutwork.com
OFFICIAL ERAS PAGE: http://www.aamc.org/students/eras/start.htm
OFFICIAL NRMP WEBSITE: http://www.nrmp.org/

SUGGESTED READING:

USMLE STEP 1

First Aid for the USMLE Step 1 : 2006 (First Aid for the Usmle Step 1) (Paperback) by Vikas Bhushan, Tao Le - $44.95
HIGH YIELD SERIES
    Gross Anatomy
    Histology

Embryology
Neuroanatomy
Physiology
Behavioral sciences
Biochemistry
Pathology
Pharmacology
Microbiology
Immunology
Genetics
Biostatistics
Acid-base balance

UNDERGROUND CLINICAL VIGNETTES

PRE-TEST

Robbins and Cotran Review of Pathology (Paperback) by Edward Klatt, Vinay Kumar- $ 39.95

USMLE STEP 2 CK

First Aid for the USMLE Step 2 CK (First Aid) (Paperback) by Tao Le, Vikas Bhushan- $44.95

HIGH YIELD SERIES

UNDERGROUND CLINICAL VIGNETTES
Medicine
Pediatrics
Obg
Surgery
Psychiatry
Blue print
Medicine
Pediatrics
Obg
Surgery
Psychiatry

Harrison's Principles of Internal Medicine: Patient Management Problems: Pre Test Self-Assessment and Review (Harrison's Principles of Internal Medicine Patient Management) (Paperback) by Alfred Jay Bollet $18.95.

USMLE STEP 2 CS

First Aid for the USMLE Step 2 CS (Clinical Skills Exam) (Paperback) by Vikas Bhushan, Tao Le, L. David Martin, Fadi Abu Shahin, Mae Sheikh-Ali -$ 39.95

USMLE STEP 3

First Aid for the USMLE Step 3 (Paperback) by Tao Le, Vikas Bhushan, Patrick O'Connell, Murtuza Ahmed
-$39.95

Swanson's Family Practice Review: A Problem-oriented Approach (Paperback) by Alfred F. Tallia (Editor), Dennis A. Cardone (Editor), David F. Howarth (Editor) Kenneth H. Ibsen (Editor).
$74.95

ERAS AND THE MATCH:

- Iserson's Getting into a Residency: A Guide for Medical Students, Sixth Edition (Paperback) by Kenneth V. Iserson
- First Aid for the Match (First Aid Series) (Paperback) by Tao Le, Vikas Bhushan, Chirag Amin, Steven Berk, Eric Collisson
- The Successful IMG: Obtaining a US Residency (Paperback) by Anagh A. Vora

GENERAL INFORMATION

The blog by Digitaldoc offers useful information on various issues concerning the USMLE and Residency

Webste:www2.blogger.com/profile/06490732171275104383

27

Frequently Asked Questions (FAQs)

Muralikrishna G

1. What if I fail the exam?
2. If I pass, can I retake the exam? I am not satisfied with my score, can I improve it?
3. How long are the scores valid?
4. Moonlighting
5. Night-float
6. Dress for visa interview
7. Should I take the Kaplan course for the USMLE exams?
8. Can I use old editions of the suggested books?
9. Should I use gold standard audio tapes for USMLE Step 2?
10. If I dont get the visa, will my Step 2 CS fee ($ 1200) be refunded?
11. Should I be careful about what I post on the internet?
12. What is categorical/preliminary and transitional?
13. What is the IVY league and which universities are they?
14. I want to do my fellowship in the US. Will I need to take USMLE?
15. What is the difference between an FMG and an IMG?
16. Should I enter the US through GRE or the Step 2 CS route?

1. WHAT IF I FAIL THE EXAM?

Failing the exam is one possibility one can never be prepared for. In the unfortunate event if you failing any of the exams, it is time to stop, rethink and refocus on what went wrong with your initial preparation. Often times, failure in the USMLE is due to a lack of understanding of the format and the nature of the exam. Although it is true that your USMLE transcript will record the failure and you may be asked by Program Directors during your interview about your failure, it does not mean the end of residency hopes. There are many examples of people before you who have failed not once, but numerous times, but still matched in competitive programs and specialties. So, don't lose hope.

2. IF I PASS, CAN I RETAKE THE EXAM? I AM NOT SATISFIED WITH MY SCORE, CAN I IMPROVE IT?

The simple answer is no. But there is one loophole, by which one's score can be improved. The validity of USMLE exam scores is seven years. So if seven years have lapsed since you have taken your Step I, your previous Step I exam score will be invalid and you will be asked to take the exam again. So, if you have got a low score in any of your USMLE exams, and wish to retake them, you have to wait for atleast seven years. But, keep in mind, that once you are ECFMG certified, you will not be eligible to take any of the exams for life.

3. HOW LONG ARE THE SCORES VALID?

The scores are valid for seven years only.

4. WHAT IS MOONLIGHTING?

Moonlighting is the process by which one can work part-time outside of residency to earn an additional income. Moonlighting can be in-house or out of hospital. Most residency programs have strict rules regarding moonlighting. Most programs have opportunities for in-house moonlighting, that does not require a state medical license, and can be done on an H-1B visa. J1 visa holders cannot moonlight under any circumstance. Moonlighting hours should not violate the work hour regulations of the ACGME. Out of hospital moonlighting usually requires written approval by the GME office, and also requires a state medical license, the requirements for which, vary state to state.

5. WHAT IS NIGHT-FLOAT?

Night-float is a rotation during residency where you exclusively work night shifts, this can vary from 5 pm to 7 am, 10 pm to 8 am, and so on. This is usually 2 to 4 weeks every year. By using a night float system, not only are residency programs able to meet the ACGME work hour regulations, but also change the call system to non-overnight.

6. HOW TO DRESS FOR VISA INETRVIEW?

This is a common question and a difficult one to answer. For men, it is simple, as you can wear a neat formal suit, with a tie, formal trousers and shoe. For women, the choice is wider, and this is discussed in the chapter on interview.

7. SHOULD I TAKE THE KAPLAN COURSE FOR THE USMLE EXAMS?

Kaplan Medical offers preparatory courses for the USMLE exams. The courses are available for USMLE Step 1, Step 2 CK, Step 2 CS and Step 3. It is a tough decision deciding whether or not to take the Kaplan course. There are people who swear by it and there are also people who swear as it. We, the authors cannot recommend for or against using the Kaplan courses.

The choice and decision about Kaplan must be individualized. However, we hope to help by listing a few relevant pros and cons.

Pros

1. Clear time frame of preparation
2. Material given at the course plus regular tests and evaluation.
3. Study partners
4. Videos for each subject
5. Small study groups
6. Well stocked library
7. Flexible hours
8. Extremely useful if there is a lapse of 2 years or more after graduation (when in a non-internal medicine residency or when not in residency).

Cons

1. Cost of roughly 55,000 for each of the steps.
2. Quite a number of aspirants have aced the exams with top scores in spite of not attending.
3. Difficulty in taking the course if you are in medical college as student or in a postgraduation course/residency despite flexible timings.
   Overall, as we said above taking Kaplan is an decision based an individual capacity be it financial or academic.

8. CAN I USE OLD EDITIONS OF THE SUGGESTED BOOKS?

Old editions can be used as long as they do not significantly compromise the quality of the content you are reading. If may be a good idea to compare the old edition to the current edition and then make a decision based on the price difference and the difference in content.

9. SHOULD I USE GOLD STANDARD AUDIO TAPES FOR USMLE STEP 2?

Gold standard tapes are available as part of preparation materials for Step 2. Again, this is an individual decision. As discussed in the chapter on Acing the USMLE Step 2 CK, except for Kaplan, rest of the materials are option and are up to the individual reader, their self-assessment of their strengths and weaknesses that should help make the decision.

10. IF I DON'T GET THE VISA, WILL MY STEP 2 CS FEE ($1200) BE REFUNDED?

Yes thankfully yes, in the worst case scenario, of you not being able to take the USMLE step 2 CS exam in the United States, due to denial of a visa to enter the United States, ECFMG offers a full refund of the Step 2 CS fees. Contact finance section of ECFMG should this situation arise.

11. SHOULD I BE CAREFUL ABOUT WHAT I POST ON THE INTERNET?

Absolutely yes. It is illegal to post-examination material on the internet. It is clearly mentioned USMLE that such irregularity will be reported in the USMLE transcript, and in some cases, also lead to revoking of the USMLE score. Be very careful what you discuss especially after the examination on public forums.

12. WHAT IS CATEGORICAL/PRELIMINARY AND TRANSITIONAL?

Transitional, preliminary and categorical are again terms confusing to many IMGs. Transitional refers to one year of rotations in various specialties (Medicine, Surgery, OBG, etc). Transitional year is usually done before doing a specialty such as Categorical surgery, dermatology, radiology, ophthalmology, etc., all which require a year of medicine before starting the particular specialty.

A preliminary year can be in Medicine or Surgery. A preliminary year is an alternative to doing transitional year. The difference between Preliminary (usually referred to as "prelim") and Transitional is that in Preliminary, you work either in Medicine or Surgery for one year, whereas in Transitional, you work in different specialties for one year.

Categorical refers to the combined three year program in Medicine or the five year program in General Surgery. By categorical, they mean "committed", meaning that these applicants are already committed to the particular specialty.

A word of caution, though. Be wary of ranking and matching in stand alone preliminary medicine or surgery programs, since you match for a prelim year, and may have nowhere to go after your prelim year.

13. WHAT IS THE IVY LEAGUE AND WHICH UNVERSITIES ARE THEY?

Ivy league is a league of universities and colleges in northeastern United States that have a reputation for scholastic achievement and social prestige. Traditionally, Ivy League institutions carry a great deal of Prestige, and are extremely competitive to get into. As an IMG, it is next to impossible to get into an Ivy League institution, especially for competitive specialties, unless you are truly exceptional.
- Brown University in Providence, Rhode Island,
- Columbia University in New York, New York,
- Cornell University in Ithaca, New York,
- Harvard University in Cambridge, Massachusettes,
- Princeton University in Princeton, New Jersey,
- Dartmouth College in Hanover, New Hamphire,
- Yale University in New Haven, Connecticut and
- The University of Pennsylvania located in Philadelphia, Pennsylvania.

14. I WANT TO DO MY FELLOWSHIP IN THE US. WILL I NEED TO TAKE USMLE?

This is a very complicated question. The answer to this depends on what your long-term plan is.

Choice A: I have completed my residency in my home country, I just want to train in the US and go back to my home country.

This is the simplest choice. If you have completed residency in your home country and want to train in a particular subspecialty in the United States, you still need to take the USMLE to be ECFMG certified. Only ECFMG certified physicians can provide patient care in the US. Once you complete your residency and are ECFMG certified, you can apply for fellowships in the US (again, personal contacts work best), and do a 1-3 year fellowship, and go back to your home country.

Choice B: I have completed my residency in my home country, but I want to settle in the United States.

This is more complicated. Here, if one wants to go into private practice in the United States, one has to be American Board (AB) certified. To be American Board certified, one has to complete a residency here in the US. So even, if you have completed your residency and fellowship in your home country, you still have to go through residency and fellowship, if you want to go into private practice in this country.

But, if one wants to go into Academic Medicine in the United States (meaning, stay as faculty in an University program), one can finish their residency in their home country, finish a fellowship here in the United States, and in exceptional cases, stay as a faculty in the University where you did you fellowship. This has been done before, but has to be approved one a case-by-case basis by the University.

15. WHAT IS THE DIFFERENCE BETWEEN AN FMG AND AN IMG?

This difference is not universally used. FMG usually refers to a non-US citizen graduating from a foreign medical school (anybody from Australia, Asia or Europe). IMG usually refers to a US citizen who went abroad for medical school. Traditionally, US citizens go to medical schools in the Caribbean or Europe and then come back to the US for residency training. Often times, Caribbean medical students do all or part of their clinical rotations in the United States. Hence IMGs start off with a distinct advantage as compared to FMGs, due to citizenship status and one to two years of US clinical experience.

16. SHOULD I ENTER THE US THROUGH GRE OR THE STEP 2 CS ROUTE?

The decision to pursue training in the US and how to go about making the decision has been discussed in detail earlier in the book. Once the decision is made, every single person, without exception, has to go through a grueling series of exams, the USMLE step 1/Step 2 CK/Step 2 CS and Step in 3 in order to get ECFMG certification and then apply for a residency.

The series of exams are interestingly designed. Although the first two steps, namely, the USMLE Step 1 and Step 2 CK can pretty much be taken anywhere in the world, the second two exams are administered exclusively in the US. Hence, one has to enter the United States to take these exams in order to be eligible for a residency. How to enter the United States is a question that is on everybody's mind and one of the most frequently asked question by US residency hopefully. Here, I will try to answer that question.

Although options like marriage, acquiring a greed card/getting a research job on a H1 visa/training as a nurse in Russia and then entering the US as a nurse/going to the United Kingdom, getting a job and then applying for a US visa from UK are options used by some residency hopefuls, for most people, the choice is between taking FRE/TOEFL, applying for a master's degree or taking the first two steps in India and then applying for tourist visa to enter the US to take the USMLE Step 2 CS.

Interestingly, the choice between F1 visa (GRE/TOEFL) vs the B1/B2 Visa (USMLE Step 2 CS) appears to vary according to geographic location and medical school, atleast in India. Most people in North India and most of Andhra Pradesh appear to take the GRE/TOEFL route, apply to US universities for master degrees like MPh/MS/Biomedical engineering/Business administration, apply for a F1 visa and enter the US. This option is considered to be safe, since the chances of rejection of a F1 visa are apparently lesser than the chances of rejection of tourist visa. The obvious disadvantages of the F1 route are the student loans acquired before residency, 2-3 years spent in programs you may not have a great interest in, and most importantly, taking a break from active, clinical medicine for a long period of time. The important issue that has come up in recent years, for IMG's applying for US residencies, is the number of years since graduation from medical. Hence doping a master's degree is a double edged sword in that an MPH/MBA/.biomedical engineering degree may strengthen your application, but at the same time weaken it owing to the years lapsed since graduation. Hence the decision must be a strictly individual one.

On the other hand, taking USMLE Steps 1 and 2 (CK) in India, applying for a tourist visa in India, and then coming to the US to take Step 2 CS/Step 3, doing an observership/elective in the US, getting letter of recommendation, and applying for residency appears to be a fairly straightforward idea. Not so. It is pretty much a well known fact that getting tourist visa in India is a dicey issue. The biggest problem being a natural tendency for Indians to move out of India is a dicey issue. The biggest problem being a natural tendency for Indians to move out of India to "greener pastures", thereby making the consular officers in the US embassies to be overtly cautions before issuing a tourist visa to Indians. But getting a multiple entry tourist visa makes things easy. One can apply for a visa when he/she is in medical school, or during residency, hence the number of years since graduation when applying for a US residency can be zero or one year, thereby making you an attractive candidate.

Overall, the choice of FRE or USMLE first is a difficult one. There are other chapters in this book that extensively discuss the details of the above two routes, and with the information provided in those chapters, and in discussion with family and friends, a decision can be made on which route to take to enter the United States for further training.

[28]
Program Director Speaks
Jayashree Sundararajan

April L McVey MD Program Director and Associate Professor, University of Kansas Medical Center, Department of Neurology.

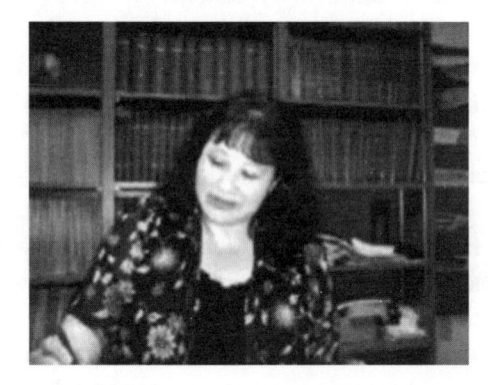

1. Know which visas are acceptable for the institution you are interviewing at. For example, at KUMC we can only take J1 visas or green card holders. We can't take people with only employment authorization cards or H1, F1 visas.
2. Speaking and writing English is important. Many of the interviewees who struggle with English are ranked lower. If shy but speak English well, demonstrate it.
3. Interviewing faculty are frequently suspicious that applicants from outside the US are trying to get into any specialty that will let them get a foot in the door. Demonstrate real interest in neurology with specific examples. Offer this even if it isn't touched upon by the interviewer.

4. I recommend bringing up in a casual way an interesting case of neurological disease that you came into contact with—that you can use to demonstrate some knowledge of neurology or neuroanatomy. Read up on it so that if questions are asked, you know what you are talking about.
5. I am impressed by enthusiasm, kindness, politeness, happiness, confidence with modesty, and sense of humor... I am not impressed by arrogance, boredom, dishonesty and someone who I have to force to get words out of them.
6. You have probably heard me say this during your interview, but certain traits are essential. Being a team player, a problem solver not a problem causer, having positive energy, enthusiasm, enjoying hard work, integrity, politeness, kindness to patients, etc.
7. Neurology residents have to read, read and read some more. It is easy to get into neurology, it is not easy to graduate a competent neurologist. Though I don't expect PG2s to have read through a neurologic textbook, I do expect them to know some basic neuroanatomy. If I knew ahead of time that someone would not spend much time studying or reading neurology, I wouldn't take them. I still have to get on some people to read (Americans and IMGs).
8. You don't have to include this one, but an attractive tidy appearance is a must! I can think of two cases of people interviewing who made a bad impression. We all have occasions when our breath is noticeable but one candidate had very bad breath. I don't think that person flossed their teeth on a regular basis or saw a dentist for a cleaning. Americans are maybe too vigilant about body odors, but when interviewing, be aware. The other person had the price tag on their suit prominently displayed. This was commented on by many people who saw that person.
9. An occasional male applicant looked at women inappropriately or said inappropriate things to them. Not to the faculty, but to female residents or support staff. This gets back to the committee.

Take what you need from my advice list. I hope there isn't anything offensive- I did try to be as honest as possible.

April L McVey MD
Associate Professor
<AMCVEY@kumc.edu>

Currently Dr. McVey serves as the Program Director for the Neurology residency program. Her clinical interests are in neuromuscular disorders, evaluation and experimental treatment, and in neurodegenerative diseases, specifically Alzheimer's Disease.

Sample Documents

Muralikrishna G and Jayashree Sundararajan

WARNING: DO NOT USE THE SAME LETTER OR DOCUMENT
SAMPLE THANK YOU LETTER

Dear Dr. Harik,

Thank you for the opportunity to interview for the PGY1 neurology position on Friday, November 4, 2005. The experience strengthened my interest in the position and reinforced my confidence in my ability to excel should I be selected.

My education and experiences so far has equipped me for this position and my enthusiasm and hardwork will ensure my success. The tour of the facilities and conversations with Dr. Ashish Nanda gave me a clear overview of the patient population and what's expected of residents at your program. Now that I have a better idea of what the position entails, I am even surer that I would be an asset to your program.

I had an opportunity to visit the Indian students association celebration of Diwali on Saturday and felt very much at home at Little Rock. I am considering your program as my first choice as it gives me and my husband to work at the same place. Little Rock promises to be an ideal destination to start our family.

I look forward to an opportunity to visit with you again and spend a day with the residents. Thank you for your time and consideration.

With warm regards,

SAMPLE PROGRAM COORDINATOR LETTER

Sample 1

Dear Ms. Treadway,

I immensely enjoyed the visit to Little Rock as well as the department of neurology on Friday, November 4, 2005. Thank you very much for putting us all at ease. I found the stay at the Hilton Inn to be very pleasant and convenient. Thank you for recommending the place for me to stay there.

I had an opportunity to visit the Indian student's association celebration of Diwali on Saturday and felt very much at home at Little Rock. I am considering your program as my first choice as it gives me and my husband to work at the same place. Little Rock promises to be an ideal destination to start our family. I look forward to an opportunity to visit with the program again. Thank you.

Sample 2

Dear Ms. Woolsey,
It was a pleasure to have met you again yesterday. When I started my search for the residency spot, the most important factor to me was to go to a place where I felt at ease, at home. I felt that the first time I visited your program and again yesterday and I am positive I would feel it every single day I am there. I am excited about the opportunities that lie ahead of me at KU. I am looking forward to joining your Department. Thank you for your confidence in me.

SAMPLE PERSONAL STATEMENT

SAMPLE OBG PERSONAL STATEMENT

When I first attended the Medical School in University of Aleppo I asked myself: "Which specialty do I want?" At that moment I could not figure out the answer. I preferred to delay making the decision until having a clear idea about the different specialties. In the first 3 years I studied the medical basics, finding them very useful and interesting in contrast to others who describe them as boring and hard subjects. Physiology, anatomy and pathology attracted me, as the latter is the most significant link between the basic and the clinical sciences. By the end of third year, I was looking forward to starting the clinical science.

My clinical years started with self-confidence derived from my feeling that I am supported by a very strong basic background. At this point I started seeking the right specialty. Even though I found all of my clinical rotations challenging I always find myself attracted towards Ob/Gyn rotations. I gave its rotation more attention by coming early to do history and physical exam, doing rounds with my attending doctors, and listening to them discussing each patient's case and analyzing every symptom and sign, in addition I have had the opportunity to work with women on the different issues they face throughout life from family planning, childbirth, cancer and surgery to menopause. During those rounds, I learned that I should educate patients and their families about their situation, and the time that I spend to build a relationship with my patient will have a positive impact on everything (diagnosis, treatment, and follow-up). However, I got a conclusion that it is the basic principle of medicine "To Be a good doctor you need more than knowing the mechanism of diseases; it requires an attention to the human side of patients and their families and this is the difference between the physician as a technician and the physician as a caring supporter". By that time I realized that Ob/Gyn is what I was seeking.

Obstetrics and Gynecology is the field of medicine which ranges from dealing with pregnancy and infertility to managing, both medically and surgically, disorders of the female reproductive tract. Yet for people like myself, it entails much more. I am the type of person who enjoys counseling, preventative care, working with my hands and being involved with intimate and personal details of the lives of my patients, THIS IS THE FIELD FOR ME!

I had the honor to participate in the Medical Productive Camp in the rural areas of Al-Hasaka city. It was one of the most exciting events in my life when the women of a small village came to us to take Hepatitis B vaccine after a lecture about Hepatitis B that I helped in organizing. I was moved by the poverty that the women of those areas faced daily and I have grown more committed to reaching out to women with unmet needs.

While I was in fourth year of my six years of medical school, I went to the UK to do 2 months of electives in the University of Cambridge in acting internship Internal Medicine. It was a great experience for me but I heard a lot about the advanced system in the US hospitals from my friends, who were members of the US medical teams, so I decided to do residency in the USA. It was like a dream but every dream can be made real by a good plan. I passed USMLE Step 1, then went to the USA to do 2 electives in Baylor College of Medicine in GI consultation and Texas Heart Institute in General and Cardiovascular Surgery. During this elective I had the honor to work with the most famous surgeons in the world, I got the chance to interact and participate in more than 75 surgical cases, it was a nice experience, and however, Ob/Gyn is still my favorite. I involved myself in the ward duties and diagnostic procedures (such as echocardiography, endoscopies, ERCP and cath lab) and stayed up late discussing cases and monitoring patients with my attending doctors. I found myself in a state of continuous learning, as each day in addition to the rounds there was a morning report and a midday lecture. I enjoyed the cooperation the team displayed, using computer to order labs and medication and checking the new updates. I became familiar with the American Medical System and I was surprised by the importance of the social worker's role. When I came back to my country I felt that my personality as a doctor became more mature.

As a member of the Medical Club of Aleppo University, I did many presentations in prenatal care, sexually transmitted diseases and Ethics. I always enjoyed teaching and interacting with students. Learning is an everyday activity to me, and I have learned not only from my attendings but also from my residents and students.

During my medical schooling I worked very hard, I graduated in April 2005 and ranked 2nd of my class. I have had the honor to be the director of the graduation ceremony 2005 which was the most beautiful ceremony during the 34 years of the Medical School history.

My goal in general is to be an obstetrician/gynecologist, and in specific, to enhance the lifestyle of women, as they don't only want to be cured but also to live happily and independently. I am looking forward to a residency-training program that will develop my clinical and technical skills, promote patient education and prevention and treat me as a part of a family. I have confidence in my abilities, enjoy working as a member of team, and feel I can be a strong advocate for my patients.

With my skills and motivation, I am looking forward to being an active member in your medical staff.

PSYCHIATRY PERSONAL STATEMENT 1

"Take up medicine. You would feel happy being able to help people everyday." My father had said when I was faced the choice of choosing engineering or medicine as my career. That was when I was 17 years old. Today I feel blessed and rewarded amply for heeding his advice. Writing this personal statement has made me to reflect on the moments in my life when I had made crucial decisions that have led me to this point in time, to seek you.

Being born in a small town—Salem, I was fortunate to be educated in one of the best convent schools in South India. I had much creative energy and I was active in the English club, writing short stories and poems. It was also then I started my first love—books. I am still a voracious reader and have come a long way since the times of Enid Blyton. Being accepted in medical school took me to one of the most prestigious schools in South India, Sri Ramachandra Medical College. All of the 5 years I spent there, every moment was special. With every clinical posting I was in awe of how perfect the human body is. Being affiliated with the Harvard University opened opportunities to participate in monthly teleconferences. Then began my musing to train at least in part in the USA.

My experiences in medical school has given me a glimpse into the hearts and lives of many, witnessing raw emotions of pity, remorse, tenderness, hatred, longing in their most dramatic forms. It made me curious as to why people do the unpredictable, the amazing sometimes crazy stuff they do. My interest in the workings of the brain and the mind continued to grow all through my clinical years. I choose to work on a project on Refsum's disease as a part of my degree in Bioinformatics. The research environment was simulating. The strides in the field of medicine seemed to have their beginnings in the laboratory. It was around that time I started to consider a career in genetics.

After graduation, in accordance with the traditions in my country, I entered an arranged marriage to a neurosurgery resident. My husband was very supportive of my dreams and aspirations. He encouraged me to explore all possibilities and I decided to take a year off from medicine and take time to see what paths lay before me. I applied for courses in hospital administration and choose Oklahoma City University. I spent summers working on getting ECFMG certified .Visiting hospitals here and volunteering time made me realize what care could be and education could be.

Earlier this year, the fateful tsunami affected Chennai among many other places. Staying so many miles from my family and coming so close to losing them, I choose to spend 6 months in India. During this time, I worked with Dr. Easwaradass in the Neurology Department. Although the complexity of science and the way it can be unraveled with mathematical precision held me in awe, it was the psychiatric components and human behavior that I was drawn to. I felt in part, it was the writer in me exploring various personalities. What I sought was a career that would enable me to indulge in my interests as well as substantially improve the lives of people. I found myself oscillating between psychiatry, neuroscience and neurogenetics.

I asses myself both as a clinician striving towards perfection and also as a person striving towards empathy for my patients. Sadly in my experiences, generally illnesses of the mind are often accompanied with stigma and people who need help, seeking it are considerably low. Personally I became aware of the true impact of coping with mental illness, when my sister was diagnosed with bipolar disorder. We found ourselves swept in the same tempest of confusion, fear and frustration, facing overwhelming loads of information. The challenges facing those afflicted are twofold with the society although changing, still stigmatic and from what science has to offer—largely underdiagnosed and a range of medications and therapy, and long term care. I am prepared to face these challenges. I want to eventually be able to make a difference in this world in not only being to treat these ailments but also participate in awareness programs about the options available and recognize more people who could be helped. I want to be able to answer questions like, could emotions and moods be predicted? What are the genetic links to personality? And many more.

At this point I see myself considering incorporating my clinical experience with research into a career in psychiatry eventually being able to focus on the genetic basis. The wide spectrum of cases and the challenges involved and being able to help in promotion of mental health reinforces my belief on my career choice of psychiatry, and I hope to contribute something original to this field. My clinical acumen, diagnostic abilities, communication skills and empathy would find full meaning here. I would feel complete and satisfied if I could break at least a fragment of the great barriers that mentally ill people face when it comes to accessing the care they require. To this I am committed.

PSYCHIATRY PERSONAL STATEMENT 2

Statement of Purpose

"The primary purpose of it all is to provide the deepest, richest, psychological and spiritual existence for the greatest number of people and the best measure of things is simply which human beings life is enhanced by what we do. Otherwise, it doesn't matter.

— Harold Taylor, Philosopher.

Early in high school, I was introduced to the concept of Maslow's hierarchy of needs. Intrigued by the idea I wanted to learn more about Maslow's theories. Eagerly, I read and pondered these novel concepts and my existential interests flourished. However, while the social sciences and humanities stimulated me creatively and intellectually, I knew I would only be fulfilled if I could use my knowledge and skills to offer meaningful service to others. I have always been interested in the questions of how sociocultural environment and psychobiological processes interact to mould a person, and how a particular sociocultural surround comes into being. Since high school I had hoped for a career in psychiatry—the field where I felt my academic, social-science/humanistic interests might be most usefully applied. And I was particularly interested in such culturally influenced illnesses as anorexia and bulimia; substance abuse and depression in adolescents.

B. Berston MD once said: "... a funny thing happens to medical students on their way to becoming physicians: they forget how to hold a conversation." I have resisted this and I believe that my ability to communicate makes me well suited to pursue a career in psychiatry. While I possess the science background necessary for success in the profession, I also consider myself a "people" person. At medical school, I have most enjoyed the courses that examine neuroscience and human behavior. I especially liked studying psychopharmacology and the biological basis of addiction and other disorders. Early lectures about developmental neuroscience impressed upon me the gravity of psychological traumas in pregnancy, infancy and childhood. During my basic science training,

I had opportunities to work with psychiatric patients. While developing my interviewing and assessment skills, I quickly realized I had a talent for listening to people's stories and learning about their cultural backgrounds. It was incredibly gratifying to see the transformation of patients impaired by their mental illness who were again functional after receiving appropriate therapy. I also enjoyed situations where I was able to help patients develop insight into their emotions and behavior during the course of their treatment. I found ample opportunities for studying psychopathology throughout my clinical rotations and was intrigued by the idea that the mind strongly contributes to the development, course, and outcome of most medical conditions. Psychiatry challenges me intellectually, gives space to my creativity, and affords me an opportunity to utilize my greatest personal traits.

Doing a Masters in Public Health (MPH) degree after Medical School has helped me to appreciate preventive mental health efforts and the role of media and culture from a different perspective. While I envision patient care as being the focus of my medical career, I plan to include advocacy and education in my professional activities. Abundant opportunities exist to educate the public and the medical community about the realities of mental illness and the need for resources. I see a great need and opportunity for expanding our understanding of etiology, course, and treatment options for mental illnesses.

My intention is to examine the process by which South Asian and American adolescents learn ways of experiencing and of behaving which help them—or fail to help them—make sense of their social realities. This will be the Special Project required for my MPH. Both the United States and India are large, multiethnic, complex societies, but with significant and provocative differences. America has been, for several generations, the epitome of an industrialized, secular society, but is only now grappling with the issues of multiculturalism. India, my home, conversely, has long accommodated ethnic and religious pluralism (with varying degrees of success), and is only now coming to terms with rapid urbanization, industrialization, and Westernization. The effect of these processes—pluralization and modernization—on individuals is only poorly understood. What is known, however, is that both processes contribute to the difficulties faced by adolescents who must negotiate their ways through social realities unknown to their parents. I am interested in a comparative study of the way South Asian and American adolescents deal with the stresses of imminent adulthood, especially as those stresses manifest themselves psychologically. In this country, these include substance abuse, eating disorders, depression, reckless behavior and so forth.

One of my strong points is expressing my ideas, and presenting them to the average layman in a comprehensible manner. I did a weekly feature for the *Times of India* on mental health that was widely read and appreciated. I can deftly use humor and analogies that people understand, rather than facts and figures, to put a point across. I also have a life outside medicine. I am an avid sports-person too. I participated in athletics, cricket and basketball during school and college and am a member of the local riding club. Sports taught me the meaning of perseverance and teamwork.

For my residency training, I hope to find a program where biological psychiatry and psychotherapy are both considered meaningful components of psychiatric training and practice and that also fosters an atmosphere of learning and encourages resident research activities. I also look forward to exposure to a diverse patient population and to the various subspecialties in psychiatry. I wish to work hard, be intellectually stimulated and challenged, and gain the proficiency I need to become an excellent clinician. I am excited at the thought of entering this fascinating profession and hope to make a meaningful contribution to my patients, to my residency program and to the psychiatric field. I see myself eventually as an academic, teaching and pursuing research on sociocultural factors in the development of mental illness, on community-based prevention and the amelioration of the same, and on incorporating qualitative understanding of patients' cultural beliefs and experience into psychiatric care.

SAMPLE INTERNAL MEDICINE PERSONAL STATEMENT

Medicine, the only profession that labors incessantly to destroy the reason for its own existence" – James Bryce (1838-1922).

The above statement eloquently emphasises the beauty of Medicine, the strife of man against disease aided by a professionals called physicians who strive to eradicate disease which is the fundamental reason for their existence. The word "Doctor" is derived from the Latin word "Doktoir" meaning teacher. It is my firm belief that a good physician should be a good teacher not only to his students but more importantly to his patients. During my eight week internal medicine internship, I was given the enviable task of teaching medical students in their first clinical year. After discussions with professor and the students themselves, I was able to structure a teaching program that began with basic sciences relevant to clinical medicine, continued with the art of History taking, the physical examination, clinical presentations culminating in assessment and feedback. This taught me more than I taught them, as I realized that good teaching must be oriented towards what the student wants and needs to know rather than what you would like to tell the students.

In the United States, I have spent two months at Hospitals and I have rotated through the outpatient clinics, hospital and Pathology departments and participated in the ward rounds and discussions. Specifically I learnt about medical coding, the essence and importance of medical documentations in the United States, issues of reimbursement and insurance that are specific to the practice of Health care in this country. I presented a topic of great interest "Efficacy of Antidepressants— Myth or Fact" based on an article in the British Medical Journal and received excellent feedback. I made a presentation of a rare case of spindle cell sarcoma at the Grand rounds. I was also given the opportunity to take detailed History and physical examination on patients. I managed to perform a four week research study on "Troponin I and Myocardial infarction" in the Pathology Department of the Hospital.

As an intern, during my rotation in the various departments of our teaching Hospital, I was a member of a team of physicians consisting of various specialties in the health care provided to each patient which taught me the foremost basis of any kind of the practice of medicine, teamwork. I learnt the judicious use of manpower, division of responsibilities and the presence of an efficient team make a big difference to the provision of health care. During my residency, I took forward to quality healthcare in your residency program to all my patients under the guidance of expert clinicians as a member of a team.

Overall, if selected, I believe that I can be an asset to the residency program with my patient care research and teaching activities. I hope to complete my residency and continue fellowship training. My foremost duty to my patients will be to serve as evidence-based provider combined with compassion and understanding for their concerns. I am eager to visit your program and will be honored to undergo my residency training in your program. I look forward to hearing from you.

SAMPLE MEDICAL STUDENT PERFORMANCE EVALUATION DEAN'S LETTER

Medical Student Performance evaluation
For
Jayashree Sundararajan
August 11, 2005

IDENTIFYING INFORMATION

Dr. Jayashree Sundararajan joined Sri Ramachandra Medical College and Research Institute during the academic year 1997-98. She was conferred the Degree of Bachelor of Medicine and Bachelor of Surgery (MBBS) on March 2004.

UNIQUE CHARACTERISTICS

A student with genuine concern and dedication, Dr Jayashree is brilliant at her work and has an outstanding academic record to her credit. During her basic sciences year she received distinction in all her courses which included Anatomy, Biochemistry, Physiology, Pathology and Microbiology. Her perseverance and dedicated efforts helped her to maintain her academic excellence through her clinical years and she was consistently placed in the top 10% of her class.

In addition to her academic work she is an active member of many college programs as well as inter-college programs and presentations. She was also involved in volunteer work with the blood donation drives and organizing screening programs for diabetes and hypertension. During her internship period she enrolled in part time classes in the field of Bioinformatics. She was deeply interested in research work and worked in several projects including "3-D modeling of the PAHX gene", Incidence of byssinosis in cotton mill workers of Coimbatore. As part of her preventive medicine classes she worked with the government primary health centers during the immunization drives for eradication of polio. Besides her academic and clinical interests she is a talented writer and has contributed many articles and short stories to the college magazine. She has also participated in tennis and cricket matches.

Medical student performance evaluation
Dr. Jayashree Sundararajan
Date of Graduation from Medical College

Was the student required to repeat or otherwise remediate any coursework during his medical education?	☐ No ☐ Yes If yes, Please explain:
Did the student's educational program contain any leave(s) of absence, extension(s), or other gap(s) or break(s), either required or voluntary?	☐ No ☐ Yes If yes, Please explain:
Was the student the recipient of any adverse actions(s) by the medical school or its parent institution?	☐ No ☐ Yes If yes, Please explain:

Academic Progress

The university currently has a pass/fail/distinction grading system during the entire course of study.

Pre-clinical/Basic science curriculum

She was an outstanding student in all the basic science disciplines earning distinction in all of her basic science courses.

Anatomy

"Dr. Jayashree always volunteered to do presentations and had a flair for teaching. Her presentations, however complex the topic was, would not lack clarity."

Physiology

"Throughout my classes, Dr. Jayashree consistently maintained herself in the first 5%. She demonstrated not only the ability to master the material quickly, but also the willingness to help other students in their understanding of sometimes difficult physiological concepts and methods".

Biochemistry

"A brilliant student, she is keenly interested in genetics. During the lecture portion of the courses she did not hesitate to ask questions and lead discussions. Dr. Jayashree values not only the academic and theoretical components of biochemistry but also the applied aspects as well. She was foremost in laboratory experiments conducted in the department".

Pathology

"During her course in the Dept of Pathology she actively took part in all clinical discussions. She made good presentations and was an eloquent speaker. She was a pleasant and motivated student with a good sense of humor."

Pharmacology

"Dr. Jayashree had a sound knowledge base and a willing learner. She would always refer to multiple textbooks and was extremely talented in asking challenging questions to the faculty".

Microbiology

"Dr. Jayashree is a keen participant in the class, with a strong desire to learn. She is an excellent student. She gave several excellent presentations. She integrated her microbiological knowledge well with her clinical work. She spent additional hours working with tuberculosis patients teaching them about the disease and the modes of transmission."

Core Clinical Clerkships and Elective Rotations

Members of the faculty have submitted the following evaluations of her clinical performance, which we include here verbatim and in chronological order. These comments are meant to address both strengths and weaknesses.

General Medicine

"As an intern Dr. Sundararajan has excellent bedside manners with pleasant manners. She interacts well with the unit and is a true team player. She maintains exemplary sensitivity, courtesy and respect for fellow students, staff and faculty. Her superiors have noted her to have admirable work ethics. She exhibits good personal clinical judgment in stressful situations…… she is service-oriented and volunteered in a number of free screening programs conducted by this institution and various organizations."

Pediatrics

"Dr. Sundararajan's clinical performance exceeded all required standards. Her record-keeping is accurate and neat. She volunteered to work with the ongoing vaccination programs and made presentations as to means by which to effectively communicate to the community about the importance of vaccinations and vaccination schedule. I found her to be compassionate, empathetic, pleasant, motivated, punctual and to have excellent fundamental knowledge and clinical judgement."

Tuberculosis and respiratory diseases

"Dr. Sundararajan participated in the ongoing study in our Department on the incidence of byssinosis in cotton mill workers in Coimbatore. She was involved in screening the cases and performing pulmonary function tests. She was a dedicated and effective research assistant. She is a mature and likable young woman".

Community Medicine

"A hard-working, promising individual, Dr. Jayashree is outstanding in relating principles and concepts of epidemiology with those of clinical medicine. She is a team player with a high degree of motivation, innovation and initiative and can accomplish her goals. Her polite, affable nature and her emotional maturity are well known and respected among her peers and the faculty as well. She was able to efficiently handle patient care at the primary level working in villages and basic health clinics. She also participated in the pulse polio program and volunteered to go into the slum areas and provide polio drops to each child and then saw to it that no child had been missed. She showed great concern for the condition of patients in rural settings".

Obstetrics and Gynecology

"Dr. Jayashree was actively involved in most operative procedures including tubal ligation, episiotomy and assisted in cesarean section, cervical tear repair. Her training also involved in the monitoring of patients in labour and has assisted/conducted deliveries. She was highly involved with the patients, explaining and educating them in simple language. She also attended well woman health camps along with her peers."

Radio-diagnosis

Dr. Jayashree is a student of distinction. She was very attentive and took the initiative to learn. She would always come on time and ask to see the procedures we do even if it were after hours. Her dedication impressed us. She was deeply interested in nuclear medicine. Her interest in the field of genetics led her to complete her training in obstetric ultrasound. She is a very skilled person and a quick learner. An impressive intern.

Emergency medicine

"Dr. Jayashree is a reliable and steadfast house officer who used her time in our Department to gain practical knowledge. She has also successfully completed basic life support class and advanced cardiac life support class. Dr. Jayashree distinguishes herself as an individual who exhibits an organized scientific approach to work, an ability to initiate, plan, organize and implement emergency procedures of varying degrees of complexity."

General Surgery

"Dr. Sundararajan is an energetic diligent intern, always courteous with a pleasant disposition. Her outpatient care was excellent to the point where patients would request to see her. She handled emergency calls cautiously but deftly. She was careful not to make hasty and erroneous decisions. She pays compulsive attention to details. She is inquisitive and has good understanding of her subjects. She assisted in major surgeries including in the transplant OT which is a privilege given to select students. She was clearly a leader among her peers and handled herself professionally yet was compassionate and insightful to the physical as well as emotional health of the patients she attended."

Psychiatry

Dr. Jayashree showed immense interest in learning about psychiatric disorders. She was keen to learn about psychosocial and cultural issues concerning patients. Her efforts to adapt her theoretical knowledge to the clinical situation were impressive. She was quick to grasp the strategies involved in psychiatric evaluation, and her interviewing skills were excellent. Her evaluation reports were systematic, meticulous and informative. Her reports revealed her deep understanding of psychological problems and their impact on people. Her calm and quiet approach had a soothing effect on her clients and, they found her presence reassuring.

Ophthalmology

"Dr. Jayashree distinguishes herself as an individual who exhibits an immaculate need for perfection with everything she does, ability to grasp knowledge along with compassion for helping the underprivileged. She involved herself in various community services including education camps about eye donation. She is an earnest student with genuine concern for patients' well being."

Otorhinolaryngology

"Dr. Jayashree is an above average intern, efficient and active participant. During her time with us she assisted in the outpatient department taking history, completing relevant physical examinations. She also actively involved herself in most operative procedures. She was a committed intern and her tenacity impressed us very much.

Summary

It has been a pleasure to have Dr. Jayashree as a student of Sri Ramachandra. An outstanding student and exceptional person, bright, articulate, personable and energetic. She is held in high esteem by her professors and peers. She possesses leadership skills beyond those of her fellow students and her ethical standards are beyond reproach. I believe Dr. Jayashree will be an outstanding physician and excel in whichever field of study she undertakes. I highly recommend her as a worthy candidate to your residency program and wish her every success in all future endeavors.

SAMPLE LETTER OF RECOMMENDATION

Dear Residency Program Director:

Dr X underwent training in the Psychiatry Department as a student from April 1, 1999 to April 30, 1999.

She showed immense interest in learning about psychiatric disorders. She was keen to learn about psychosocial and cultural issues concerning patients. Her efforts to adapt her theoretical knowledge to the clinical situation were impressive. She was quick to grasp the strategies involved in psychiatric evaluation, and her interviewing skills were excellent. Her evaluation reports were systematic, meticulous and informative. Her reports revealed her deep understanding of psychological problems and their impact on people. Her calm and quiet approach had a soothing effect on her clients and, they found her presence reassuring. In addition, Dr X's pleasing personality enabled her to interact freely and coordinate effectively with other members of the mental health team.

She was hard-working and was keen on updating her knowledge on psychiatric disorders. Her presentations at departmental meetings were thought-provoking. She was sincere and committed in her work. Her dedication to enhance patient care was total. She managed patients under supervision with ease, and was able to employ appropriate psychopharmacological and psychotherapeutic effectively.

Summarizing, Dr X is highly skilled and dedicated to her work. She would certainly prove to be an excellent physician at any institution she joins.

Sincerely yours,

SAMPLE MEDICAL COLLEGE TRANSCRIPT

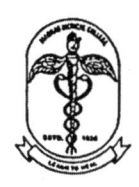

**MADRAS MEDICAL COLLEGE
AND
GOVT GENERAL HOSPITAL,
CHENNAI - 600 003. TAMIL NADU, INDIA.**

Prof JAMES PANDIAN MS MCh (Plastic),
Dean

DEAN'S LETTER FOR DR X

This is to certify that Dr X underwent the MBBS Course at the Madras Medical College, Chennai – 3 affiliated to the Tamil Nadu Dr MGR Medical University, from August 1999 to February 2005.

He has successfully completed the Compulsory Rotatory Residential Internship at Government General Hospital attached to Madras Medical College, Chennai- 3 for a period of One Year from March 2004 to February 2005.

His academic record is good. His conduct and character are good.

DEAN

Date:
Official Seal:

**MADRAS MEDICAL COLLEGE
AND
GOVT GENERAL HOSPITAL,
CHENNAI - 600 003. TAMIL NADU, INDIA.**

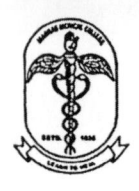

OFFICIAL TRANSCRIPT – MEDICAL CURRICULUM

This is to certify that **Dr X** underwent his MBBS Course from August 1999 to February 2005 in this College. During this period he had undergone training in the subjects shown below for the duration shown against each. Clinical instruction was given in the hospital wards and outpatient clinics under guidance.

Sl.No.	Course	Hours of Instruction
1	Anatomy, Embryology, Histology, Neuroanatomy	740
2	Anesthesia	50
3	Biochemistry	200
4	Cardiology and Cardiothoracic Surgery	25
5	Chest Medicine, Tuberculosis	10
6	Dental Surgery	25
7	Dermatology, Leprosy and Std	30
8	Diabetology	25
9	Endocrinology	5
10	Forensic Medicine, Legal and Ethical Issues, Toxicology	100
11	Gastroenterology	10
12	Geriatric Medicine	10
13	Human Sexuality and Sexually Transmitted Diseases	25
14	Medicine and Intensive Care	750
15	Microbiology, Parasitology and Immunology	300
16	Neurology and Neurosurgery	50
17	Obstetrics and Gynecology	500
18	Ophthalmology	150

Contd...

Contd...

19	Orthopaedic Surgery	150
20	Otorhinolaryngology	100
21	Pathology	300
22	Pediatrics,	150
23	Pharmacology	300
24	Physical Medicine and Rehabilitation	50
25	Physiology	600
26	Plastic Surgery	10
27	Preventive Medicine, Public Health, Nutrition, Biostatistics, Family Medicine	200
28	Psychiatry, Alcoholism, Chemical Substance Dependency and Behavioral Science	30
29	Radio Diagnosis, Radiotherapy, Radiation Safety	30
30	Rheumatology	10
31	Surgery	600
32	Therapeutics	300
33	Tropical Medicine	50
34	Urology	10

DEAN

Date:
Official Seal:

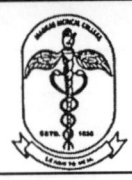

MADRAS MEDICAL COLLEGE
AND
GOVT GENERAL HOSPITAL,
CHENNAI - 600 003. TAMIL NADU, INDIA.

CERTIFIED STATEMENT OF MARKS

This is to certify that the following is a Statement of Marks obtained by **Dr X** during his Undergraduate Course of Study for the degree of MBBS, conducted by the Tamil Nadu Dr MGR Medical University.

Subjects	Marks Awarded	Date of Passing
FIRST MBBS Period Aug'99 to Aug'00 Reg. No: 1199075		
Anatomy	284 / 400	Aug '00
Physiology	307 / 400	Aug '00
Biochemistry	304 / 400	Aug '00
SECOND MBBS Period Sep'00 to Jan'02 Reg. No: 1199075		
Pathology	282 / 400	Jan '02
Microbiology	308 / 400	Jan '02
Pharmacology	299 / 400	Jan '02
Forensic Medicine	142 / 200	Jan '02
FINAL MBBS *Part-I* – Period Feb '02 to Jan '03 Reg. No: 1199075		
Community Medicine	267 / 400	Jan '03
Ophthalmology	143 / 200	Jan '03
Otorhinolaryngology	154 / 200	Jan '03
FINAL MBBS *Part II* – Period Feb '03 to Jan '04 Reg. No: 1199075		
General Medicine	365 / 500	Jan '04
Surgery	394 / 500	Jan '04
Obstetrics and Gynecology	355 / 500	Jan '04
Pediatrics incl. Neonatology	158 / 250	Jan '04

(Aggregate includes Theory, Oral, Practical, Terminal Assessment, Day to Day evaluation)

DEAN

Date:
Official Seal:

MADRAS MEDICAL COLLEGE
AND
GOVT GENERAL HOSPITAL,
CHENNAI - 600 003. TAMIL NADU, INDIA.

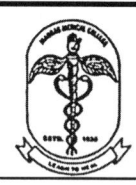

CERTIFICATE OF NON-CLINICAL CLERKSHIP
AUGUST 1999 TO JANUARY 2002

This is to certify that **Dr X** was a bonafide student of MBBS Course at Madras Medical College, during the period August 1999 to January 2002 and has undergone Non-clinical Clerkship in this Institution as follows:

Sl. No.	Course	Period of instruction From	To	Supervising professor
1.	**ANATOMY** (Anatomy, Embryology & Histology of Upper & Lower Limbs, Abdomen, Pelvis & Perineum, Head & Neck, Thorax, Nervous System)	Aug '99	Aug '00	Prof. Esther Revathy, MS,
2.	**PHYSIOLOGY** (General & Cellular Physiology Circulation, Gastrointestinal, Renal, Endocrine, Metabolism Cardiovascular, Respiratory, Special senses and Neurophysiology)	Aug '99	Aug '00	Prof. Vijayalakshmi KP, MD,
3.	**BIOCHEMISTRY**	Aug '99	Aug '00	Prof. Ebenezer MD,
4.	**PATHOLOGY** (General Pathology & Hematology, Systemic Pathology)	Sep '00	Jan '02	Prof. Taralakshmi MD,
5.	**MICROBIOLOGY** (General Microbiology, Immunology & Parasitology, Systemic Bacteriology, Virology, Mycology & Applied Microbiology)	Sep '00	Jan '02	Prof. Vijayalakshmi TS MD,

Contd...

Contd...

| 6. | **PHARMACOLOGY & THERAPEUTICS** | Sep'00 | Jan '02 | Prof. Parvarthavathini MD, |
| 7. | **FORENSIC MEDICINE** | Sep'00 | Jan '02 | Prof. Tahira Begum MD, |

DEAN

Date:
Official Seal:

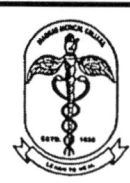

MADRAS MEDICAL COLLEGE
AND
GOVT GENERAL HOSPITAL,
CHENNAI - 600 003. TAMIL NADU, INDIA.

CERTIFICATE OF CLINICAL ROTATIONS – FIRST CLINICAL YEAR
AUGUST 2000 TO JANUARY 2002

To certify that **Dr X** has done his MBBS Course from August 1999 to January 2004 and has completed rotation in the following disciplines as part of the MBBS course.

Sl. No	Clinical Discipline	Hospital/ Location	Dates of Clerkship	Head of the Department/ Supervising Professor
1.	Obstetrics and Gynecology Including Family Planning.	Institute of Obstetrics and Gynecology, Chennai-10	09.10.2000- 22.10.2000	Prof. Gajalakshmi Subramaniam, MD, DGO
2.	Social and Preventive Medicine including Public Health.	Govt. Gen. Hospital. Chennai-3	23.10.2000- 19.11.2000	Prof. Murugan, MD, DPH
3.	General Medicine including Expenditure to Laboratory Medicine and Infectious diseases.	Govt. Gen. Hospital. Chennai-3	20.11.2000- 31.12.2000	Prof. Bennet, MD
4.	General Surgery including Expenditure to Dressing and Anesthesia.	Govt. Gen. Hospital Chennai-3	01.01.2000- 11.02.2001	Prof. T Gunasagaran, MS, MCh
5.	Dermatology	Govt. Gen. Hospital. Chennai-3	12.02.2001- 18.02.2001	Prof. Janaki MD
6.	Sexually Transmitted Diseases—Venereology	Govt. Gen. Hospital. Chennai-3	19.02.2001- 25.02.2001	Prof. Balasubramaniam, MD
7.	Ear, Nose and Throat	Govt. Gen. Hospital. Chennai-3	26.02.2001- 25.03.2001	Prof. Pacifica Simon, MS, DLO
8.	Obstetrics and Gynecology including Family Planning	Institute of Obstetrics and Gynecology, Chennai-10	26.03.2001- 22.04.2001	Prof. Gajalakshmi Subramaniam, MD, DGO

Contd...

Contd...

9. Social and Preventive Medicine including Public Health	Govt. Gen. Hospital. Chennai-3	23.04.2001- 20.06.2001	Prof. Murugan, MD, DPH
10. Ophthalmology	Regional Institute of Ophthalmology, Egmore, Chennai-8	21.06.2001- 18.07.2001	Prof. Jayalakshmi, MS, DO
11. Pediatrics including Social Pediatrics	Institute of Child Health, Egmore, Chennai–8	19.07.2001- 01.08.2001	Prof. Rama Devi, MD, DCH,
12. Tuberculosis and Chest Medicine	Govt. Gen. Hospital. Chennai-3	02.08.2001- 15.08.2001	Prof. AS Natarajan, MD, DTM
13. Psychiatry	Govt. Gen. Hospital. Chennai-3	16.08.2001- 29.08.2001	Prof. Sathyanathan, MD, DPH
14. Orthopedics including Expenditure to Rehabilitation and Physiotherapy	Govt. Gen. Hospital. Chennai-3	30.08.2001- 26.09.2001	Prof. Motilal, MS, D Ortho
15. Obstetrics and Gynecology including Family Planning	Institute of Obstetrics and Gynecology, Chennai-10	27.09.2001- 24.10.2001	Prof. Gajalakshmi Subramaniam, MD, DGO
16. General Medicine including Expenditure to laboratory Medicine and Infectious Diseases	Govt. Gen. Hospital. Chennai-3	25.10.2001- 21.11.2001	Prof. Bennet, MD
17. General Surgery including Expenditure to Dressing and Anesthesia.	Govt. Gen. Hospital. Chennai-3	22.11.2001- 19.12.2001	Prof. T Gunasagaran, MS, MCh

DEAN

Date:
Official Seal:

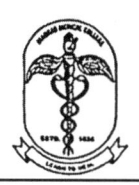

MADRAS MEDICAL COLLEGE AND GOVT GENERAL HOSPITAL, CHENNAI - 600 003. TAMIL NADU, INDIA.

CERTIFICATE OF CLINICAL ROTATIONS – SECOND CLINICAL YEAR FEBRUARY 2002 TO JANUARY 2003

To certify that **Dr X** has done his MBBS Course from August 1999 to January 2004 and has completed rotation in the following disciplines as part of the MBBS Course.

Sl. No	Clinical Discipline	Hospital/Location	Dates of Clerkship	Head of the Department / Supervising Professor
1.	General Surgery including Expenditure to Dressing and Anesthesia	Govt. Gen. Hospital Chennai-3	08.02.2002- 21.02.2002	Prof. T Gunasagaran, MS, MCh
2.	Ophthalmology	Regional Institute of Ophthalmology, Egmore, Chennai-8	22.02.2002- 07.03.2002	Prof. Jayalakshmi, MS, DO
3.	Casualty	Govt. Gen. Hospital. Chennai-3	08.03.2002- 21.03.2002	Prof. Shanthakumar, MD
4.	Radiology	Govt. Gen. Hospital. Chennai-3	22.03.2002- 04.04.2002	Prof. J Daniel, MD
5.	Dermatology	Govt. Gen. Hospital Chennai-3	05.04.2002-	Prof. Janaki, MD, DD
6.	Sexually Transmitted Diseases—Venereology	Govt. Gen. Hospital Chennai-3	12.04.2002- 18.04.2002	Prof. Balasubramaniam, MD,
7.	Ear, Nose and Throat	Govt. Gen. Hospital. Chennai-3	19.04.2002- 02.05.2002	Prof. Pacifica Simon, MS, DLO,
8.	Dentistry	Tamil Nadu Govt. Dental College, Chennai-3	03.05.2002- 16.05.2002	Prof. Thulasingam, MDS,

Contd...

Contd...

9. Orthopedics including Expenditure to Rehabilitation and Physiotherapy	Govt. Gen. Hospital Chennai-3	17.05.2002-28.06.2002	Prof. Motilal, MS, D Ortho
10. Obstetrics and Gynecology including Family Planning	Institute of Obstetrics and Gynecology, Chennai-10	29.06.2002-26.07.2002	Prof. Gajalakshmi Subramaniam, MD, DGO
11. General Medicine including Expenditure to Laboratory Medicine and Infectious diseases	Govt. Gen. Hospital Chennai-3	27.07.2002-23.08.2002	Prof. TS Kannan, MD
12. Pediatrics including Social Pediatrics	Institute of Child Health, Egmore, Chennai-8	24.08.2002-20.09.2002	Prof. Rama Devi, MD, DCH
13. Ear, Nose and Throat	Govt. Gen. Hospital Chennai-3	21.09.2002-18.10.2002	Prof. Pacifica Simon, MS, DLO
14. Ophthalmology	Regional Institute of Ophthalmology, Egmore, Chennai-8	19.10.2002-15.11.2002	Prof. Jayalakshmi, MS, DO
15. Social and Preventive Medicine including Public Health	Govt. Gen. Hospital Chennai-3	16.11.2002-13.11.2002	Prof. R. Murali, MD, DPH

DEAN

Date:
Official Seal:

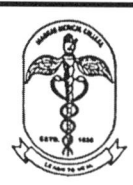

MADRAS MEDICAL COLLEGE
AND
GOVT GENERAL HOSPITAL,
CHENNAI - 600 003. TAMIL NADU, INDIA.

CERTIFICATE OF CLINICAL ROTATIONS – THIRD CLINICAL YEAR
FEBRUARY 2003 – JANUARY 2004

To certify that **Dr. X** has done his MBBS Course from August 1999 to January 2004 and has completed rotation in the following disciplines as part of the MBBS Course.

Sl. No.	Clinical Discipline	Hospital/ Location	Dates of Clerkship	Head of the Department / Supervising Professor
1.	General Medicine	Govt. Gen. Hospital, Chennai-3	17.06.03-16.08.03, 29.11.03-26.12.05	Prof. L Pari, MD
2.	General Surgery	Govt. Gen. Hospital, Chennai-3	31.03.03-02.06.03, 02.10.03-30.10.03	Prof. N Dorairajan, MS
3.	Orthopaedic Surgery	Govt. Gen. Hospital, Chennai-3	02.06.03-16.06.03	Prof. K Anbazhagan, MS, DOrtho
4.	Obstetrics and Gynecology	Institute of Obstetrics and Gynecology, Chennai-10	22.01.03-30.03.03, 31.10.03-28.11.03	Prof. Shakuntala Barathi, MD, DGO
5.	Pediatrics	Institute of Child Health, Egmore, Chennai-8	02.09.03-01.10.03	Prof. Rama Devi, M.D, DCH
6.	Dermatology	Govt. Gen. Hospital, Chennai-3	17.08.03-23.08.03	Prof. Janaki, MD, DD
7.	Psychiatry	Govt. Gen. Hospital, Chennai-3	24.08.03-01.09.03	Prof. Sathyanathan, MD

DEAN

Date:
Official Seal:

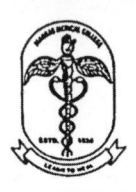

MADRAS MEDICAL COLLEGE
AND
GOVT GENERAL HOSPITAL,
CHENNAI - 600 003. TAMIL NADU, INDIA.

CERTIFICATE OF COMPLETION OF
COMPULSORY ROTATORY RESIDENT INTERNSHIP (CRRI)
FEBRUARY 2004- FEBRUARY 2005

This is to certify that Dr. X has passed the Final MBBS Examination, the Tamil Nadu Dr. MGR Medical University held in December 1998 and has worked as a Compulsory Rotatory Resident Internee for a period from Jan 1999 to Jan 2000 in the departments as detailed below:

Sl. No.	Clinical Discipline	Hospital/ Location	Dates of Clerkship	Head of the Department /Supervising Professor
1.	General Medicine	Govt. General Hospital, Chennai-3	29.11.04-13.12.04, 29.12.04, 15.01.05-28.02.05.	Prof. L Pari, MD
2.	General Surgery	Govt. General Hospital, Chennai-3	16.03.04-30.03.04, 15.04.04-23.04.04, 09.05.04-30.05.04	Prof.R. Anbazhagan, MS
3.	Orthopaedic Surgery	Govt. General Hospital, Chennai-3	31.03.2004- 14.04.2004	Prof. K Anbazhagan, MS, D Ortho
4.	Obstetrics and Gynecology	Kasturba Gandhi Hospital for Women, Chennai-5	31.05.2004- 20.06.2004	Prof. Shakuntala Barathi, MD, DGO
5.	Primary Health Centers National Control Programme	Govt. General Hospital, Chennai-3	15.09.2004- 28.11.2004	Prof. R. Murali, MD
6.	Community Pediatrics	Institute of Child Health, Egmore, Chennai-8	31.08.2004- 14.09.2004	Prof. Vasantha Mallika, MD, DCH
7.	Casualty and Trauma	Govt. General Hospital, Chennai-3	30.12.04-07.01.05	Prof. Ramani, MD

Contd...

Contd...

8.	Maternal and Child Health & Family Planning	Kasturba Gandhi Hospital for Women, Chennai-5	21.06.2004-30.07.2004	Prof. Shakuntala Barathi, MD, DGO
9.	IMCU	Govt. General Hospital, Chennai-3	08.01.2005-14.01.2005	Prof. C Rajendran, MD
10.	Elective 1 (Psychiatry)	Govt. General Hospital, Chennai-3	31.07.2004-14.08.2004	Prof. Sathyanathan, MD, DPH
11.	Elective 2 (Radio diagnosis)	Govt. General Hospital, Chennai-3	15.08.2004-30.08.2004	Prof. TS Swaminathan, MD
12.	Pediatrics	Institute of Child Health, Egmore, Chennai-8	14.12.2004-28.12.2004	Prof. Vasantha Mallika, MD, DCH
13.	Ophthalmology	Regional Institute of Ophthalmology, Egmore, Chennai-8	24.04.2004-08.05.2004	Prof. Jayalakshmi, MS, DO
14.	Otorhinolaryngology	Govt. General Hospital, Chennai-3	01.03.2004-15.03.2004	Prof. Balasundaram, MS, DLO

DEAN

Date:
Official Seal:

Index

A

Acing the USMLE step 1 32
  subjectwise preparation 35
    anatomy 35
    behavioral sciences 36
    biochemistry 36
    microbiology 37
    pathology 38
    pharmacology 38
    physiology 35
    question banks and consolidated sources 39
  time-table for preparation 34
  what are the subjects tested 32
  what study materials to use 33
Acing the USMLE step 2 CK (clinical knowledge) 41
  question banks and consolidated sources 45
  subjectwise preparation 42
    ethics/biostats 44
    medicine 42
    OG 43
    padiatrics 44
    psychiatry 44
    surgery 43
  time-table for preparation 42
    a tentative schedule 42
    as for revision 42
  what are the subjects tested 41
  what study materials to use 42
Acing the USMLE step 3 65
  time-table for preparation 67
  what are the subjects tested 66
  what study materials to use 66
Applying to programs—individualising curriculum vitae and personal statement 149
  application process: Curriculum vitae 149
  application process—personal statement 150
Applying to universities in the US 88

B

Behavioral sciences 36
Book for internal medicine residency 151

C

Combining a masters program and USMLE 92
Competitiveness of specialty 148

D

Difference between an FMG and an IMG 224
During residency in specialty 151
  book for internal medicine residency 151
  life during internal medicine residency 151

E

Exam day strategies 27
Exam: GRE, GMAT and TOEFL 83

F

Family practice 168
  competitiveness of specialty 169
  non-competitive specialty 169
  during residency in specialty 170
  rank order list 169
  salary profiles and lifestyle issues 170

G

General information 218
Getting the F1 visa 90
Gold standard audio tapes for USMLE step 2 222
Green card processing 122

H

Harrison's manual of medicine 184
How do I prepare for the USMLE 24

I

Internal medicine 147
  by choice or by chance 147
International test delivery surcharge 24

Interviewing in specialty 151
   internal medicine residency interview 151
Ivy league 223

J

J1 vs H1 visa 124
John's Hopkins manual 184

K

Kaplan course for the USMLE exams 221

L

Links to courses 216

M

Medical specialty as an IMG 118
   how to select a specialty 119
   which specialty 118

N

NBME scores 26
Neurology 189
   applying to programs—individualising curriculum vitae and personal statement 189
     Alabama 190
     Arizona 190
     Arkansas 191
     California 191
     Illinois 191
     Indiana 191
     IOWA 191
     Kentucky 191
     Louisiana 191
     Michigan 191
     Minnesota 191
     Missouri 191
     New York 192
     North Carolina 192
     Ohio 192
     Oklahoma 192
     Oregon 192
     Pennsylvania 192
     South Carolina 192
     Tennessee 192
     Texas 193
     Virginia 193
     Washington 193
     Wisconsin 193
   competitiveness of specialty 189
   interviewing in specialty 194
     interview 194
     rank order list 194
       preparing rank order list 194
     salary profiles and lifestyle issues 195
     specialisation after residency 195
Nuts and bolts of residency application 125
   by August of year before match 127
     observership 127
     research the programs 127
   chronological time frame 126
   interview season: Nov/Dec/(Jan) of year preceding the match 133
     few or no interview what to do 139
     how to prepare for the interview 135
     how to travel to the interview 134
     questions that you can ask 138
     scheduling the interviews 134
     selection criteria for interviews for an FMG 133
     what to do when you receive the interview call 133
   July of year preceding match 126
   June of year preceding match 126
   match week 142
   NRMP registration 133
   post match scramble 142
   pre-match offer 141
     advantages 141
     disadvantages 141
   rank order list deadline 141
     submit ROL (rank order list) 141
   September 1 of year preceding match 132
     apply 132
     how many programs to apply 132
   timelines and deadlines 125
   USMLE step 3 exam 133

O

Obstetrics and gynecology 172
   Alabama 175
   applying to programs—individualising curriculum vitae and personal statement 173
   Arizona 175
   California 175
   competitiveness of specialty 173
   Connecticut 175
   during residency in specialty 181
     during Ob/Gyn residency 181
     PGY-1 181

Index

PGY-2 182
PGY-3 182
PGY-4 182
Florida 175
Georgia 175
Illinois 175
Indiana 175
interviewing in specialty 177
   evaluate a specific residency program 179
   guidelines for Ob/Gyn residency interview 177
Massachusetts 176
Michigan 176
New Jersey 176
New York 176
North Carolina 176
Ohio 176
Pennsylvania 177
personal statement 174
   guidelines for soliciting letters of recommendation 174
rank order list 180
   match day 180
   preparing final match list 180
salary profiles and lifestyle issues 187
   Ob/Gyn lilfestyle 188
   obstetrician-gynecologists (Ob-Gyn) earn in USA 187
South Carolina 177
specialisation after residency 185
   academics 186
   going back home 187
   private practice 185
   subspecialty/fellowship training in obstetrics/gynecology 186
Virginia 177
Washington 177
West Virginia 177
Official websites 215
Old editions of the suggested books 221
Other competitive specialties 205
   list of other specialties 205
      general rules to get into competitive specialties 205
Other routes of entering the United States 96
   F2/J2/H4 dependents 97
   green card 97
   marriage 97

P

Pediatrics 156
   applying to programs—individualizing curriculum vitae and personal statement 156
   applying to programs 156
   competitiveness of specialty 156
   interviewing in your specialty 157
   interview 157
   rank order list 158
   salary profiles and lifestyle issues 159
   specialisation after residency 158
Pre-exam day strategies 27
Psychiatry 160
   applying to programs–individualising curriculum vitae and personal statement 161
   competitiveness of specialty 161
   during residency in specialty 167
   specialisation after residency 167
   interviewing in your specialty 165
   interview 165
   rank order list 167
      preparing rank order list 167
   salary profiles and lifestyle issues 167

R

Rank order list 151
Research before residency 101

S

Sample documents 228
Sample letter of recommendation 242
Sample medical student performance evaluation dean's letter 236
   identifying information 236
   unique characteristics 237
      academic progress 238
      community medicine 240
      core clinical clerkships and elective rotations 239
      emergency medicine 240
      general medicine 239
      general surgery 240
      obstetrics and gynecology 240
      ophthalmology 241
      otorhinolaryngology 241
      pediatrics 239
      pre-clinical/basic science curriculum 238

psychiatry 241
radio-diagnosis 240
tuberculosis and respiratory diseases 239
Sample personal statement 229
psychiatry personal statement 1 231
psychiatry personal statement 2 233
sample internal medicine personal statement 235
statement of purpose 233
sample OBG personal statement 229
Sample program coordinator letter 227
Specialisation after residency 152
after the internal medicine residency 152
Specialties 117
competitive 117
non-competitive 117
Student visa (F1) 83
Study partner 26
Surgery 196
applying to programs—individualising curriculum vitae and personal statement 198
making the decision 198
competitiveness of specialty 197
during residency in specialty 200
surgery—preliminary and categorical 200
surgical residencies malignant and exploitative of the IMGs 203
surgical residencies take longer time to finish 203
rank order list 200
salary profiles and lifestyle issues 204
specialization after residency 204

T

Three steps of the USMLE 16
To dress for visa interview 221
Tourist visa (B1/B2) 77
preparing for the interview 80
documents 79
on the day of interview 80
some common questions 80
preparing the documents 78
visa application forms 78
procedure to book an appointment 78
before getting visa appointment 78
to get visa appointment 78
types of a tourist visa 77

U

UK: A closed door for IMGS 6
clinical attachments 7
cracking the PLAB 6
current trends and employment prospects 6
passing in IELTS 6
traditional route for PG medical training in UK for IMGs 6
ultimate decision making process 10
Underground clinical vignettes 217
United States clinical experience (USCE) 107
doing research and presentations 109
how to get letters of recommendation 109
medical graduate 107
how to get an observership 107
medical student 107
what to do during the observership 108
which places offer observership 110
USMLE mission statement 16
USMLE step 2 CS high yield notes 55
list of cases commonly tested in the exam 62
abdomen 63
CNS 62
CVS 63
joints 63
Ob/Gyn 63
pediatrics 63
psychiatry 64
skin 64
telephone conversation 64
sample case sheet to be used in the exam 55
abdominal exam 57
mental status exam 55
neuroexam 56
respiratory system 56
thyroid exam 58
what to do in each station 58
past history 59
present history 59
sexual history 61
social history 61

Index

USMLE step 2 CS how to prepare 47
  consolidated sources and forums 54
    cons 54
    pros 54
  exam center, travelling, scheduling and standardised patients 50
    center locations 50
    choosing the exam center 50
    results 52
    standardized patients 52
    travelling to the test center 51
  general tips 53
    plan a for step 2 CS 53
  what are the subjects tested 47
  what study materials to use 48
USMLE step 3: High yield notes 69
  100 golden rules for CCS cases 69
USMLE steps 26

W

What to do during observation 108